AF527903

Looking Back
Looking Forward

Looking Back, Looking Forward

A Profile of Sexual and Reproductive Health in India

Edited by
SHIREEN J. JEJEEBHOY

Rawat Publications
Jaipur and New Delhi

Population Council
New Delhi

ISBN 81-7033-879-4
© Population Council, New Delhi 2004

No part of this book may be reproduced or transmitted in any form or by any means, electronic or mechanical, including photocopying, recording or by any information storage and retrieval system, without permission in writing from the publishers.

Published by
Prem Rawat for *Rawat Publications*
Satyam Apts., Sector 3, Jawahar Nagar, Jaipur 302 004 (India)
Phone: 0141 265 1748 / 7006 Fax: 0141 265 1748
E-mail: info@rawatbooks.com
Website: www.rawatbooks.com

Delhi Office
4858/24, Ansari Road, Daryaganj, New Delhi 110 002
Phone: 011-23263290

Typeset by Rawat Computers, Jaipur
Printed at Chaman Enterprises, New Delhi

Contents

List of Tables and Figures

Tables

Figures

Abbreviations

AIDS	acquired immune deficiency syndrome
ARV	anti-retroviral
ART	assisted reproductive techniques
CBO	community-based organisation
CT	*Chlamydia trachomatis*
GC	gonorrhoea
HbsAg	hepatitis B surface antigen
HIV	human immunodeficiency virus
HPV	human papilloma virus
HSV	herpes simplex virus
IVF	*in vitro* fertilisation
IEC	information, education and communication
ICDS	Integrated Child Development Services
ICPD	International Conference on Population and Development
IUD	intra-uterine device
IVF	in vitro fertilisation
MSM	men having sex with men

MTP	medical termination of pregnancy
PNDT	pre-natal diagnostic techniques
NPP	National Population Policy
NACO	National AIDS Control Organisation
NFHS	National Family Health Survey
RCH	reproductive and child health
RTI	reproductive tract infections
STD	sexually transmitted disease
STI	sexually transmitted infection
TV	*Trichomonas vaginalis*
WHO	World Health Organisation

Foreword

Over the last decade, India has made significant advances in meeting the sexual and reproductive health needs of and enabling the exercise of informed choice by females, males and young people. Contraceptive targets were abolished and there has been a movement towards decentralised and client-centred services and respect for community needs. In the National Population Policy of 2000, the government reiterated its commitment to ensuring voluntary and informed choice, enhancing quality of care, providing access to the full package of sexual and reproductive health services and extending the reach to all. The Reproductive and Child Health Programme (phase 1), launched in 1997, has put in place, at the field level, the goal of comprehensive and client focused services that enable the exercise of informed choice. The HIV/AIDS programme has now been integrated with reproductive and child health at the primary health care level. The needs of young people and the need to involve men more fully within the purview of sexual and reproductive health programmes have been strongly articulated. Measures have been taken to ensure gender equity, equality and to enable women to exercise greater control over their sexual and reproductive health.

Looking Back, Looking Forward: A Profile of Sexual and Reproductive Health in India provides a thoroughly researched and fair review of where we stand, in 2004, with regard to our commitment to meeting the sexual and reproductive health needs of women, men and young people. Its chapters cover a range of sexual and reproductive health concerns, including contraceptive use dynamics, maternal and newborn health, infertility, abortion, reproductive tract and sexually transmitted infections (STIs) and young people's situation and needs. The review highlights achievements made, as well as both socio-cultural and programmatic impediments to the attainment of sexual and reproductive health. Gender issues are highlighted in every chapter and the focus on domestic violence underscores gross persistent inequities. Cross cutting each chapter are programmatic commitments and achievements; they reveal that much has been accomplished but a lot remains.

As we move towards ICPD+10, this volume is a useful reference that describes, through a careful review of available evidence, the extent to which policy and programme level changes have been accompanied by changes in the sexual and reproductive well-being of people. It highlights the fact that progress has not been equal on all fronts. On the positive side, infant mortality has declined, access to skilled attendance at delivery has increased and unmet need for contraception has been reduced. Yet, the report suggests that there is a long way to go: maternal mortality continues to be unacceptably high, the spread of STIs including HIV is worrisome and wide gender imbalances and limited exercise of reproductive rights continue to be experienced by large segments of the population, particularly women. The needs of young people (aged 10-24) who represent some one third of our population, remain poorly understood and served. Despite the Medical Termination of Pregnancy Act (MTP), lack of access to safe services results in millions of women resorting to unsafe abortion. Other disquieting trends are also noticed. The misuse of pre-natal diagnostic techniques to identify the sex of the foetus and the consequent abortion of female foetuses is one such trend. In short, it concludes, as have we in the Ministry of Family Welfare, that although this last decade has witnessed impressive strides in some aspects of sexual and reproductive health, much remains to be done.

The report, authored by researchers of the Population Council India and co-published by the Population Council India and the World Health Organisation's South East Asia Regional Office (SEARO) is essential reading for policy makers, programme implementers in government and non government sectors, rights advocates and researchers alike. It provides a succinct assessment of what we have achieved and where we have failed and a strong empirical assessment upon which policies and programmes should be based.

As we take stock of the events of the decade since ICPD, this synthesis of what we have achieved and the outstanding challenges is not only timely, but also informative and thought provoking.

Prasanna Hota
Secretary
Department of Family Welfare
Ministry of Health and Family Welfare
Government of India

7 June 2004

Acknowledgements

This book provides a comprehensive review of various dimensions of the reproductive health and rights situation in India, ranging from the concerns of young people to the magnitude and patterns of reproductive tract and sexually transmitted infections from a review of the available literature. We hope that the evidence and recommendations contained in this book will highlight major programmatic challenges and at the same time inform the design and content of policy-relevant empirical research on sexual and reproductive health in India.

The review was supported by generous financial support from WHO/SEARO, which we gratefully acknowledge. In particular we would like to express our deep appreciation to Dr Monir Islam, Director, Family and Community Health Department, WHO/SEARO and Dr Ardi Kaptiningsih, Regional Advisor for Reproductive Health and Research, WHO/SEARO for encouraging the Council to undertake this activity, and for their guidance and support throughout the course of the project.

As the book shows, this has been a collaborative effort of a team of colleagues from the Population Council, India. Team members contributed at every stage of the project—from conceptualising the book and issues to be highlighted, to undertaking a thorough perusal of the literature, to preparing comprehensive draft working papers that not only describe the situation but also provide a critical overview of each theme. This book is a testimony to their commitment and enthusiasm.

This review would have been impossible without the insights, cooperation and support of many. Each draft working paper benefited from the comments and suggestions of a number of reviewers. We are grateful to Leena Abraham, Dinesh Agarwal, Rama Baru, Surinder Jaswal, Ardi Kaptiningsih, Arvind Mathur, Veera Mendonca, Suneeta Mittal, A.R. Nanda, Madhubala Nath, Saroj Pachauri, Vikram Patel, T.K. Roy and Leela Visaria for their valuable comments and suggestions. Their insights and comments, incorporated in the text, have helped shape the focus of the book and enriched the contributions.

Each draft working paper was then summarised to highlight major issues pertaining to each topic and it is these extended summaries that are reproduced in this publication. For turning the collection of papers into a cohesive volume, we acknowledge the significant contribution of Deepika Ganju. Deepika worked with Council staff to structure the book, and in the process not only reworked contributions to fit the format of a consolidated volume, but also provided, for each chapter, valuable technical review and suggestions for modification. Her significant editorial and technical contributions and careful attention to detail have made the volume more readable and precise and we are hugely indebted to her for these.

The administrative requirements involved in the production of this book cannot be under-estimated. Komal Saxena and Asha Matta have ably supported the production of the book in many ways, from accessing literature to preparing the manuscript to finalising references and their assistance in ensuring the quality of this book is gratefully acknowledged.

This project could not have been completed without the support and encouragement of Dr. Saroj Pachauri, Regional

Director, South and East Asia, Population Council. As authors, we are grateful to her for sharing her insights on the sexual and reproductive health situation in India.

I would like to end by expressing, on behalf of all authors, our appreciation to the Population Council and all of its staff members, who helped in small and big ways in making this book possible.

Shireen J. Jejeebhoy
Population Council,
New Delhi

June 2004

Part I

Setting the Stage

Setting the Stage

Shireen J. Jejeebhoy, K.G. Santhya, Ravi K. Verma, Leila Caleb Varkey, Vaishali Sharma Mahendra, Anjali Widge, Vijaya Nidadavolu, Deepika Ganju

The last decade has witnessed momentous and multi-dimensional changes in the sexual and reproductive health situation in India. The policy and programme environment has undergone a significant shift from a narrow target-oriented family planning approach to a broader orientation that stresses sexual and reproductive health and the exercise of reproductive rights more comprehensively. Over the same period, there have also been major changes in the context of sexual and reproductive health. Some changes, such as declining infant mortality, increased access to skilled attendance at delivery, and declining unmet need for contraception have been positive. Other trends are extremely disturbing, such as stagnating levels of maternal mortality, the spread of sexually transmitted infections (STIs) notably HIV, the persistence of wide gender imbalances and limited exercise of reproductive rights by large segments of the population, particularly women. The decade has raised concern about the unique sexual and reproductive health needs of the young, a group whose needs remain poorly understood and served. It has seen the absorption of new technologies into everyday sexual and reproductive life, such as new methods of contraception and pregnancy termination, the misuse of pre-natal diagnostic techniques for sex selection, and increasing and poorly regulated access to assisted reproductive techniques (ARTs). Finally, while the need for a rights-based approach has been recognised, this has not been reflected in terms of government's accountability in the realisation of health rights, implementing legislative and judicial reforms, providing adequate support services and promoting a supportive environment for vulnerable groups. In short, despite the strides made on several fronts, India continues to face a situation of considerable sexual and reproductive ill health and lack of informed choice.

While over the course of the 1990s, several studies have addressed aspects of sexual and reproductive health in India, there remains a need to synthesise the lessons learned, identify achievements and obstacles, and outline strategies and actions to enhance sexual and reproductive health in the 21st century. In this endeavour, a first step is the compilation of a profile on the current situation and an assessment of the needs in India in this sector. The objective of this book is to provide a comprehensive review of various dimensions of the reproductive health and rights situation in India, ranging from the concerns of young people to the magnitude and patterns of reproductive tract infections (RTIs) and STIs, from a review of the available literature. We hope that the evidence and recommendations in this book will highlight major programmatic challenges and at the same time inform the design and content of forthcoming policy-relevant empirical research on sexual and reproductive health in India.

We start with a few words to guide the reader. In conducting this synthesis, we have cast a wide net, exploring the published and grey literature available on each aspect of sexual and reproductive health in the country. We have found that the evidence continues to be incomplete and patchy: for example, while evidence on the patterns of contraceptive use is not only comprehensive but also available at national and sub-national levels, evidence on other topics—infertility, RTIs and STIs, risk-taking behaviours of adolescents to name a few—comes from small scale studies whose findings may not be generalisable to the population at large. What we do know suggests considerable state-wise heterogeneity in levels and patterns of prevalence, in access to services and in socio-cultural, gender and health system determinants. Each chapter highlights these regional disparities and the need for flexible policies and programmes. In the following sections, we explore such issues as the sexual and reproductive health situation of young people; contraceptive use dynamics; pregnancy-related health and care; the context of induced abortion; reproductive tract and sexually transmitted infections, including HIV; the infertility situation; and gender-based violence. Certain cross-cutting issues—gender double standards and power imbalances, exercise of informed choice, male involvement, quality of care and services, for example—are central to each topic and have been addressed within the discussion of each subject rather than as separate sections. A certain amount of overlap is thus inevitable and we argue that this should be retained in order that each topic is addressed as thoroughly as possible.

In this introduction, we provide the background in which sexual and reproductive health and choice are experienced. We focus on four over-arching themes, notably, the socio-cultural context, the absorption of new technologies into sexual and reproductive life, the programme situation and changing policy environment, and public health organisation and infrastructure. We also review health sector reform initiatives in the country.

Socio-cultural setting

India's population, which crossed one billion in 2000, is characterised by a sex ratio that continues to be unfavourable to females, a large rural population, heavy reliance on agriculture and widespread poverty with significant proportions living below the poverty line. Some current demographic and reproductive health indicators are reflected in Table 1.

Table 1

Selected demographic and reproductive health indicators

Sex ratio, 2001 (females/1,000 males)[1]	933
Child sex ratio, 2001 (0-6 years)[1]	927
Infant mortality rate (1994-98)[2]	67.6
Total fertility rate (1996-98)[2]	2.85
Young Women	
Women aged 20-24 married by 18 years, 1998-99 (%)[2]	50
Estimates of premarital sexual activity among females 15-24 years (%)[3]	0-9
Estimates of premarital sexual activity among males 15-24 years (%)[3]	15-30
Married adolescents 15-19 years using contraceptives (%)[2]	8
Contraceptive Use Dynamics[2]	
Contraceptive prevalence rate	48
Unplanned pregnancies (%)	21
Currently married women with an unmet need (%)	16
Sterilised women as a proportion of all couples using modern methods (%)	71
Currently married couples using male or couple-dependent methods (%)	10
Maternal Health and Care[2]	
Maternal mortality ratio (per 100,000 live births)	540
Neonatal mortality rate, 1994-98	43
Skilled attendance at delivery (%)	42
Women receiving all recommended antenatal services (%)	20
Non-institutional births receiving a check-up within two months postpartum (%)	17
Induced Abortion	
Prevalence range for sex-selective abortions (%) (community-based studies)[4]	3-17
Maternal deaths resulting from unsafe abortion, 1998 (%)[5]	9
Estimated number of total abortions (million)[6]	6.7
Estimated number of abortions at approved centres (million)[7]	0.6
Infertility	
Women aged 40-49 years currently married estimated to be childless (%)[2]	3.8

Contd...

Contd...

Sexually Transmitted Infections (STIs)	
Estimated new STI infections annually (million)[8]	40
Estimated new HIV infections annually, 2001 (million)[9]	0.11
People who seek STI services in the public sector (%)[8]	5-10
People who are aware that consistent condom use prevents HIV transmission (%)[10]	59
HIV prevalence range among antenatal women, 2001[9]	0-1.75
HIV prevalence range among STD clinic patients, 2001[9]	0-26.6
Domestic Violence[2]	
Ever married women beaten by husbands (%)	19

Note: For definitions, see text.

Sources: (1) RGI, 2001; (2) IIPS and ORC Macro, 2000; (3) Jejeebhoy, 2002; (4) Elul et al., 2003; Ganatra et al., 2000; Khanna, 1997; Malhotra et al., 2003; (5) RGI, 2000; (6) Chhabra and Nuna, 1994; (7) Khan et al., 1999; (8) NACO, 1998; (9) NACO, 2003a; (10) NACO, 2001a

A brief overview of socio-demographic characteristics of the population drawn from the National Family Health Survey (NFHS) (IIPS and ORC Macro, 2000) suggests that:

- The infant mortality rate is currently 68/1,000 and the under-five mortality rate 95/1,000. Achieving the national socio-demographic goal of an infant mortality rate of below 30 per 1,000 live births by the year 2010 remains a challenging task.
- Access to services is limited. Only 37 per cent of rural women live in a village with a primary health centre or subcentre; 80 per cent and 45 per cent live in villages with a primary and middle school, respectively; and 43 per cent live in villages with a post-office.
- A significant proportion of the population remains illiterate and wide geographic and gender disparities in enrolment—particularly middle and secondary school enrolment—persist. For example, while 15 per cent of young males aged 15-19 are illiterate, over twice this proportion (32 per cent) of females are illiterate. And while 58 per cent of young males aged 15-17

are enrolled in school, only 40 per cent of young females are. Only 44 per cent of women aged 15-49 had completed primary education compared to 69 per cent of men.

- As far as housing characteristics are concerned, 40 per cent have no electricity, 64 per cent have no toilet facility, 38 per cent do not have access (within 15 minutes) to safe drinking water and two in three homes are *kuccha* or semi-*pucca*. A composite index of standard of living compiled by NFHS suggests that a low standard of living characterises over one-third (36 per cent) of all Indian households.

It is well recognised that in patriarchal settings such as India, hierarchical gender relations and unequal gender norms impact women's sexual and reproductive health and choice and act as significant obstacles to access services and facilities. Equally, the achievement of good sexual and reproductive health may be inhibited by such structural factors as poverty and malnutrition, early marriage and inadequate educational and health systems. Although there are regional variations with women in the south facing somewhat fewer constraints than those in the north, undoubtedly women in both regions are far less empowered to have a say in their own lives than are men. From an early age, gender role differentials persist: compared to adolescent boys, females have limited autonomy and face huge constraints on decision making, mobility and access to resources. Double standards ensure that young females are closely supervised as their chastity is inextricably linked to the family's honour (both natal and marital). At the same time, daughters are viewed as a 'source of misery' and a drain, through dowry, on the family's resources, while a son is 'the saviour of the family'. After marriage, a young woman is expected to remain largely invisible and under the authority of her husband's family. She has little say in domestic decisions and little freedom of movement. Almost the only avenue available to enhance her prestige and even security in her husband's home is through her fertility, and particularly the number of sons she bears. Women who have borne only daughters can be subjected to harassment, and childlessness can be grounds for divorce or abandonment.

Gender roles have significant implications for sexual and reproductive health and choice. Gender norms condone early onset of sexual activity, pre- and extra-marital casual sexual relations and sex worker contacts among young males while severely proscribing even the hint of sexual misconduct among young females. Lack of awareness, lack of spousal intimacy and communication on sexual matters, and widespread gender-based violence compound women's inability to negotiate safe sex, seek appropriate health care or experience a healthy pregnancy. Finally, gender roles that perpetuate the 'culture of silence' inhibit women from communicating a health problem or seeking prompt treatment unless it inhibits them from carrying out their daily chores. This 'culture of silence' is even more pronounced for gynaecological and reproductive morbidity that are so closely linked with sexuality.

New technologies

The last decade has witnessed the incorporation of new technologies into sexual and reproductive life in several ways. New methods of contraception such as the CopperT-380A have been introduced into the programme, enabling protection for a period of 10 years, and injectables are currently available in the private sector. The introduction of innovative abortion technologies, such as the improved manual vacuum aspiration technique, is expected to increase the availability of safe abortion services. Emergency contraception has also become available, enabling the user to avoid unintended pregnancy if used within 72 hours of unprotected sex.

In 2002, medical abortion was approved by the Drug Controller of India as a method for inducing abortion, and local manufacture of mifepristone and misoprostol is under way (Coyaji, 2002). Although not yet incorporated into the programme, it is widely available over-the-counter. The technology has considerable promise as it is non-invasive, affordable, easy to use, safe, effective and requires a relatively uncomplicated infrastructure. It does not involve hospitalisation and thus allows for greater independence, control and privacy for women. At the same time, there is concern that the very fact that it is easy to use may lead to its misuse, and many have called for caution in expanding its accessibility, noting the need for client counselling, appropriate medical backup, well trained providers, appropriate medical supervision and clear guidelines for use.

Several studies have confirmed that sex-selective abortion has become so widespread in parts of India that it has distorted the sex ratio at birth (Retherford and Roy, 2003; RGI, 2001). In the large majority, it is female foetuses that are aborted. While the practice is particularly pronounced in settings in which son preference is especially strong, there is evidence that the practice is well-known, cutting across all socio-economic sub-populations, and in many cases, is unsafe.

Finally, ARTs have become increasingly accessible. While these offer hope for the infertile, they also have potential adverse health consequences. ART services are largely market-driven, and like sex detection centres, a number of private centres offering ART have emerged. Quality of care remains, however, of significant concern: inadequate information and counselling are provided, informed consent procedures are unsatisfactory, success rates are low, and services are both expensive and highly commercialised. Like pre-natal diagnostic techniques, there is concern about the misuse of this technology, including its role in enabling pre-natal sex detection. Recognising the need for effective regulation, the Indian Council for Medical Research has recently issued guidelines for the regulation of ART clinics (ICMR and NAMS, 2002).

Policy and programme environment

Over the course of the 1990s, existing policies and programmes in the area of sexual and reproductive health have undergone significant changes, and new policies and programmes to address hitherto underserved population groups and neglected issues have been introduced. These include, notably, the National Population Policy 2000, the Reproductive and Child Health Programme, the Tenth Five-year Plan (2002-07), the National Youth Policy 2000 (draft) and the National AIDS Prevention and Control Policy 2002. Additionally, legislative measures in the area of sexual and reproductive health have been introduced such as the amended Medical Termination of Pregnancy (MTP) Act, 2001 and the Pre-natal Diagnostic Techniques (Regulation and Prevention of Misuse) (PNDT) Act, 1994. Also currently under discussion is the proposed Protection from Domestic Violence Bill, 2001. The extent to which these programmes have been implemented in practice and have succeeded in empowering vulnerable communities and individuals to gain access to care and exercise reproductive rights remains, however, unclear.

We provide here a broad overview of the main policies and programmes; details are presented in later chapters.

National Family Planning Programme

The National Family Planning Programme was launched in 1951 with the demographic objective of reducing birth rates to the extent necessary to stabilise population at a level consistent with the requirements of the national economy. During the first decade of its existence, family planning was considered more a mechanism to improve the health of mothers and children than a method of population control (Visaria, 2000; Visaria and Chari, 1998). Clinic-centred family planning service delivery, along with health education activities, were promoted during this period.

The Third Five-year Plan period (1961-66) marked a subtle shift in programme emphasis, from the welfare of women and children to the macro objective of population stabilisation (Visaria and Chari, 1998). An extension-education approach replaced the original clinic-centred approach and the programme was integrated with existing health services during this period. During 1965-75, the programme was integrated with the maternal and child health programme, and at the same time, time-bound method-specific targets for population control were introduced. As is well known, the target-oriented approach became highly coercive during the period of the Emergency (1975-77). The backlash of the coercive approach compelled subsequent governments to stress the voluntary nature of the family welfare programme. In the 1980s, the time-bound, target oriented approach was revived with greater emphasis on promoting reversible methods and measures for child survival. As a part of the strategy, incentive payments for acceptors and motivators of contraceptive methods were vigorously promoted (Visaria, 2000).

The 1990s witnessed dramatic changes in the family welfare policy and programme in the country. The passing of the 72nd and 73rd Constitutional Amendments and Panchayati Raj and Nagar Palika Acts in 1992, set in motion the process of democratic decentralisation, and brought the family planning programme, legally, into the domain of *panchayati raj* institutions. In addition, several factors including the stagnation in the family planning programme, organised pressure from multiple constituencies to address issues of quality and choice and the recognition of inherent constraints in the programme contributed to changes in policy approach (Visaria, Jejeebhoy and Merrick, 1999). An additional catalyst was provided by the International Conference on Population and Development (ICPD) in 1994 and the Beijing Women's Conference in 1995. In 1996, the government took the radical decision of eliminating method-specific contraceptive targets that had been used to guide, monitor and evaluate the programme for decades, replacing it with what was initially called the Target-free Approach, where goals are set at the community level rather than determined at the Centre. In 1997, the Target-free Approach was recast as the Community Needs Assessment Approach, and a decentralised participatory planning system was put in place.

Reproductive and Child Health (RCH) Programme

The Reproductive and Child Health Programme, which was launched in 1997, focuses on the principles of client satisfaction and utilising and upgrading the existing health infrastructure to deliver high quality health services. It seeks to integrate services for the prevention and management of unwanted pregnancy, promotion of safe motherhood and child survival, and the prevention and management of RTIs and STIs. The programme aims to expand services to meet the needs of hitherto under-served and neglected population groups, including adolescents, economically and socially disadvantaged groups such as urban slum and tribal populations. To make the programme a people's programme, the new approach champions local need-based, decentralised, participatory planning and monitoring, and seeks to involve several stakeholders in more meaningful ways to move the new agenda forward (MOHFW, 1997).

The new approach represents a dramatic change in the culture of the family welfare programme (Pachauri, 1999), and for the first time, the programme has focused attention on gender concerns. It seeks to address gender issues impinging on women's health by improving quality of care, including the interaction between providers and clients; increasing the availability of female health care providers at the primary health care level; addressing neglected concerns of women such as RTIs; addressing the needs of neglected population sub-groups like adolescents; organising gender sensitisation training for stakeholders; encouraging male involvement in reproductive health; and facilitating women's and men's involvement in monitoring reproductive and child health through client feedback (World Bank, 1997). Presently (late 2003), components of the second wave of the Reproductive and Child Health Programme are being finalised.

National Population Policy (NPP) 2000

The National Population Policy, adopted in February 2000, further legitimised the paradigm shift. In May 2000, the National Population Commission was set up to guide the translation of policy rhetoric into programmes. The National Population Policy provides a policy framework for achieving the twin objectives of population stabilisation and promoting reproductive health within the wider context of sustainable development. Several state governments have framed state-specific population policies, broadening the scale of policy discourse.

The immediate objectives of the National Population Policy are to address the unmet need for contraception and health system personnel, and to provide integrated service delivery for basic reproductive and child health care. By 2010, the National Population Policy aims to achieve infant mortality rates below 30 per 1,000 live births, a maternal mortality ratio below 100 per 100,000 live births; school drop-outs at primary and secondary levels below 20 per cent; 80 per cent institutional deliveries; 100 per cent deliveries by trained personnel; and 100 per cent registration of vital events. In the medium term, the National Population Policy expects to achieve the goal of bringing the total fertility rate to replacement level by 2010 through vigorous implementation of inter-sectoral operational strategies (MOHFW, 2000).

The National Population Policy has delineated twelve strategic themes to achieve these objectives, including decentralised planning and implementation, convergence of service delivery at the grassroots, empowering women and encouraging male involvement, meeting the unmet need for family welfare services, addressing the needs of disadvantaged and under-served population groups and forging public-private partnerships.

The National Population Policy affirms the government's commitment to the provision of quality services, information and counselling, and expanding contraceptive method options in order to enable people to make voluntary and informed choices. Disincentives have not been included in the National Population Policy, though several promotional and motivational measures are to be implemented at the community and individual level. Unlike in the past, these incentives are not just for sterilisation but have been linked to the level of poverty, delayed marriage, antenatal and delivery care, birth registration, the birth of a girl child and immunisation (Pachauri, 2000). However, it is a cause of concern that some of the policies adopted by the states are diametrically opposed to the principles of equity and equality espoused by the National Population Policy. In their urgency to reduce population growth, some states have articulated several open or 'veiled' disincentives, such as debarring individuals who marry before the legal age at marriage from seeking jobs, getting admission in educational institutions and applying for loans, or debarring individuals with more than two children from contesting local body elections (Government of Madhya Pradesh, 2000; Pachauri, 2001). These policies will negatively affect women who hardly play a role in deciding the age at which they are married or the number of children they bear (Qadeer, 2000). In some cases, the implementation of the two-child policy may lead to an increase in sex-selective abortions (Buch, 2003).

National STD and AIDS Control Programme and Policy

The National STD Control Programme was initiated in 1946 (before India's independence) and remained operational until 1991. However, the programme was weak both in terms of content and implementation. Following reports of the first HIV case in the mid-1980s and the emerging HIV/AIDS epidemic, the National AIDS Control Programme was launched in 1987. In the initial years, the programme focussed on raising public awareness, screening of blood for transfusion and conducting surveillance activities in the epicentres of the epidemic (NACO, 2002b). Recognising the synergy between STIs and HIV/AIDS, in 1992, the National STD Control Programme was integrated with the National AIDS Control Organisation (NACO) (NACO, 1998). The National AIDS Control Project was launched in the same year. The thrust of the project has been on changing behaviour through interventions, particularly among high-risk groups, supporting decentralised service delivery and protecting human rights by encouraging voluntary counselling and testing and discouraging mandatory testing (NACO, 2003a).

The National AIDS Prevention and Control Policy 2002 envisages effective containment of the infection levels of HIV/AIDS in the general population in order to achieve zero-level of new infections by 2007 (NACO, 2002b). To meet these objectives, the policy has delineated various strategies including raising awareness, controlling STIs, ensuring the safety of blood and blood products, improving services for the care and support of people living with HIV/AIDS, and creating an enabling socio-economic environment. The policy reflects the paradigm shift currently under way, and emphasises the importance of inter-sectoral coordination, forging partnerships with multiple stakeholders including NGOs and community-based organisations, decentralised planning and implementation, and integration of services. It recognises that the HIV/AIDS must be seen not only as a public health issue but also as a problem of development.

Tenth Five-year Plan (2002-07)

The Tenth Five-year Plan has identified a number of targets that have implications for reproductive health. It outlines efforts in three broad areas: (a) meeting the unmet need for contraception; (b) reducing infant and maternal mortality; and (c) enabling families to achieve their reproductive goals. Eleven targets that can be monitored are defined and include a reduction in (a) the decadal growth rate of population from 21.3 per cent in the period 1991-2001 to 16.2 per cent during the period 2001-11; (b) the infant mortality rate from 68 to 45 by 2007 and 28 by 2012; and (c) the maternal mortality ratio from 407 per 100,000 live births to 200 by 2007 and 100 by 2012. At the same time, efforts have been targeted towards addressing the unmet need for maternal and child health and contraception, particularly in states where mortality and fertility declines have been lagging. Issues such as RTIs and STIs, adolescent reproductive health, unintended pregnancy and access to safe abortion are also addressed. Finally, the Plan focuses on the health infrastructure and the need to focus on improving quality of care, strengthening pregnancy and newborn health services, improving immunisation coverage against vaccine preventable diseases; promoting inter-sectoral coordination, especially with the Integrated Child Development Services (ICDS) programme; and improving the coverage and quality of health care for vulnerable and under-served adolescents. Such issues as counselling, access to and provision of good quality services and follow up care are emphasised.

Draft National Youth Policy 2000

The draft National Youth Policy 2000, addresses the needs of those aged 13 to 35, and stresses the need for a multisectoral approach to youth, with a thrust on 'youth empowerment,' notably education, skill building and leadership as well as nutrition, and equality of opportunity. While it discusses the need for access to health services among young people, especially women, and cites the need for reproductive health 'guidance,' population and family life education, its obvious focus lies on nutrition and education, rather than on sexual and reproductive health matters.

Medical Termination of Pregnancy (MTP) and Pre-natal Diagnostic Techniques (Regulation and Prevention of Misuse) (PNDT) Acts

The Medical Termination of Pregnancy (MTP) Act was passed in 1971 and came into effect in 1972. The Act enables trained practitioners to terminate a pregnancy of less than 20 weeks duration in several conditions, including risk to the life of the pregnant woman or grave injury to her physical or mental health, contraceptive failure, rape, and risk to the child. The Act was amended in 2002 to decentralise the approval process for registration of MTP centres and increase access to MTP services at the primary health care level.

In order to curb the trend towards sex-selective abortion following pre-natal diagnostic techniques, the Pre-natal Diagnostic Techniques (Regulation and Prevention of Misuse) Act was passed in 1996. This Act attempts to regulate the administration of pre-natal diagnostic techniques (including sonography) and the conditions under which these can be used, and prohibits communication of the sex of the foetus should the investigations be conducted. As the Act was ineffective in preventing sex-selective abortions, it was amended in 2002 to incorporate regulation of pre-conception and pre-implantation procedures for sex selection, regular recording of procedures and empowering local authorities to ensure compliance.

Health care infrastructure

Health services in India are available through the public sector, the private sector and the not-for-profit voluntary sector. The government is the primary source of preventive services such as immunisation and family planning while the private sector is largely involved in the delivery of curative care.

The public sector health care infrastructure has been developed as a three-tier system based on population norms. At the grassroots level, subcentres serve a group of villages. Primary health centres provide the next level of care, acting as referral units for six subcentres and serving as the first point of contact between the community and a medical officer. Community health centres, at the next level, serve as a referral for four primary health centres. District hospitals, located in urban and peri-urban settings, constitute the apex health care facility.

According to norms set by the government, each rural subcentre should cover a population of 5,000 in the plains and 3,000 in hilly or tribal areas. Corresponding norms for primary health centres and community health centres in the plains and hilly areas are 30,000 and 20,000, and 120,000 and 80,000, respectively (MOHFW, 2003a). While there has been considerable expansion and strengthening of the health care infrastructure, yet, in practice, access to and availability of services remain significant issues of concern. Gaps remain in infrastructure, staff, equipment, and supplies and, according to the population norms, the existing infrastructure is inadequate (MOHFW, 2003a). A recent survey of health facilities across the country reports that most facilities are not adequately staffed—almost one in ten primary health centres is functioning without any doctor, 82 per cent do not have a female medical officer and only 3 per cent are providing services for the medical termination of pregnancy (IIPS, 2001b).

The private sector, which includes providers from the formal, informal, the not-for-profit and for-profit sectors who are not directly financed by the state, and indigenous medical practitioners, has expanded in recent years. A majority of clients seek care outside of the public sector for a wide range of curative services. For example, estimates suggest that the majority of clients with symptoms of possible RTIs seek care outside public sector services, and only 5-10 per cent of those with STIs visit a public sector facility (NACO, 1998). It is not only the economically wealthy who seek private medical care; the poor also choose private providers for a variety of reasons and for a range of services.

Despite the size and complexity of the private sector in India, its general structure, functions, and the number of practitioners and facilities are unclear. In many cases, both the public and private sectors are staffed by the same practitioners—a survey of physicians found that among those employed in the public sector, 81 per cent also worked in private practice (Chawla, 1996). However, unlike the public sector, the functioning of the private sector is largely unregulated and market-driven. There is a felt need for some degree of control through the establishment of regulatory systems to ensure standardisation of service delivery by the private sector.

Health sector reform and its implications for reproductive health

As a response to current trends towards globalisation and structural adjustment processes, attention is now being paid to health sector reforms. As mentioned earlier, despite a large network of public health facilities, delivery of services in the public sector is unsatisfactory. Public spending on health in India has remained low, stagnating at around 1 per cent of gross domestic product (World

Bank, 2002). Data on public spending on health care both at the Central and state levels reveal a declining trend since 1991 (World Bank, 2002). Private spending on health, on the other hand, accounts for more than 80 per cent of all health spending and nearly all private spending is out-of-pocket making users extremely vulnerable (World Bank, 2002). Concerns about the reach and quality of the public health system in addressing health care needs have been raised and the need to develop alternative mechanisms to ensure delivery of equitable and appropriate health services has been expressed.

The direction and nature of health sector reform are largely undefined. Supported mainly by World Bank initiatives, the reform process remains a set of ad hoc experiments, mostly in the form of 'projects,' which lack a systems perspective (Baru, 2003; Nanda, 2002). Key concepts and terminologies that characterise the discourse on health sector reform in India include decentralisation, alternative financial mechanisms (such as health insurance/user's fee) to provide equitable and improved health care services, accountability, a greater role for local bodies to monitor the provision of health services, and enhanced participation of the private sector in the provision of health care services at all levels. Recent programmes and policies recognise the need for health sector reform. The Tenth Five-year Plan (2002-07) for example clearly outlines the need for evolving, implementing and evaluating different models of health care financing at the individual, family, institution and state levels. As one of the efforts towards decentralisation, the Plan emphasises the need to devolve responsibilities and funds to panchayati raj institutions.

Central and state initiatives have recently been introduced to attract private sector participation in health care. Concessions have been made in the allotment of land and investment allowances for medical equipment. In most cases, these incentives have led to the construction of large super-specialty hospitals and diagnostic facilities by large corporate houses in urban areas. Providing concessions to the private sector has not however resulted in the provision of effective reproductive health services for a larger number of rural people. It has instead led to greater choice and better quality services for the urban rich (World Bank, 2002). Moreover, the expansion of the health insurance industry has not matched the boom in facilities due to the slow process of liberalisation in the insurance sector. Besides, the vast majority of people work in the unorganised sector in rural areas, which is difficult to cover through such measures.

States such as Andhra Pradesh, Kerala, Maharashtra and Tamil Nadu are experimenting with managing primary health services in collaboration with private or semi-private partners as a contingency for World Bank loans. Several strategies have been adopted. In Tamil Nadu, some health facilities are administered by the state while the development of infrastructure is financed by private partners. In Delhi, Rajasthan, Punjab and Himachal Pradesh, some services at teaching hospitals are being contracted out to private agencies. Uttar Pradesh is employing part-time private female doctors on contract to meet the need for such providers in remote primary health centres. Kerala has set up hospital development committees within panchayats to manage funds and is experimenting with user fees. Many states now allow private pharmacies, laboratories and blood banks to function within or near hospitals where supplies and equipment are in short supply.

India's experience with health system reforms is as yet limited. Though there have been some attempts at devolution, experience shows that stakeholders at the community level may not have adequate skills to optimise resources and services to suit local needs (Ramanathan et al., 2003). It is still too early to assess the impact of these initiatives on reproductive health outcomes.

Moving ahead

As we have seen from the above discussion, the context of sexual and reproductive health in India has been evolving rapidly over the past decade. As preparations for Reproductive and Child Health Programme-2 are under way, this is an opportune moment to take stock of the continuing obstacles and barriers impeding the achievement of improved reproductive health outcomes. In the following chapters, we review specific issues related to sexual and reproductive health. Each of the issues is discussed in greater depth in later chapters. Collectively they profile the state of sexual and reproductive health that needs to be addressed and suggest related programme strategies and research requirements.

Part II

Issues and Evidence

Contraceptive Use Dynamics

K.G. Santhya

Over the decades, contraceptive use has been increasing in India. At the same time, there is a substantial unmet need for contraception. The contraceptive scenario is also characterised by the predominance of non-reversible methods, limited use of male/couple-dependent methods, substantial levels of discontinuation, and negligible use of contraceptives among both married and unmarried adolescents. As will be seen in the following discussion, there are wide regional variations in all these aspects.

The contraceptive scenario

Nationally, nearly one-half of currently married women (48 per cent) were using some method of contraception in 1998-99 (IIPS and ORC Macro, 2000). Contraceptive prevalence varied widely among states, from less than 30 per cent in Bihar, Meghalaya and Uttar Pradesh to more than 60 per cent in Delhi, Haryana, Himachal Pradesh, Kerala, Punjab, Maharashtra and West Bengal. Data for the 1990s, as reflected in NFHS 1 and 2, indicate that

---

This chapter is an abriged version of a working paper by K.G. Santhya titled 'Changing Family Planning Scenario in India: An Overview of Recent Evidence' (2003).

current contraceptive use increased by 18 per cent nationally (IIPS and ORC Macro, 2000). There has been an overall increase in contraceptive use in almost all states, except Goa, Jammu and Kashmir, and Meghalaya over the same period.

Method mix

Since the sixties, the family welfare programme has in theory adopted a 'cafeteria approach' whereby clients are provided with a choice of contraceptive methods. However, it is well documented that, until recently, the programme emphasis remained skewed towards promoting non-reversible methods, particularly female sterilisation. Nationally, female and male sterilisation together account for 84 per cent of current contraceptive prevalence due to modern methods and 75 per cent of overall contraceptive prevalence (IIPS and ORC Macro, 2000). Although reported by a negligible minority, sterilisation was the most common method used even among married adolescents, and a review of data on contraceptive behaviour of adolescents in Asian countries shows that India is the only country where such a pattern prevails (Pachauri and Santhya, 2002a). The predominance of sterilisation is observed in almost all states; more than 90 per cent of modern contraceptive method users are sterilised in all the southern states and Bihar; the situation is most skewed in Andhra Pradesh, where 97 per cent of all modern method users are sterilised. Exceptions include Delhi, Punjab and a few north-eastern states where fewer than three in five users of modern methods are sterilised.

Officially sponsored spacing methods (oral contraceptive pills, intra-uterine device [IUD] and condoms) account for 14 per cent of current contraceptive use. The use of traditional contraceptive methods is reportedly low, accounting for 10 per cent of current contraceptive use in the country.

Direct evidence on the use of male methods is scarce as men have been excluded from most of the national surveys, and small-scale studies exploring the contraceptive behaviour of men are limited. Nationally, data based on the responses of currently married women show that one in ten currently married 'couples' were using male/couple-dependent contraceptive methods (condoms, vasectomy, withdrawal and periodic abstinence) in 1998-99, which translates into 21 per cent of total current contraceptive prevalence (IIPS and ORC Macro, 2000). The data also show that the use of male/couple-dependent methods was as low 2 per cent of currently married couples in Bihar, Mizoram and Karnataka, and as high as 23-28 per cent of currently married couples in Delhi, Punjab and West Bengal.

Data specifically on the use of modern male methods show that only a small minority of currently married couples were using such methods (condoms 3 per cent and vasectomy 2 per cent). Condom use was typically low in almost all the states, except Delhi and Punjab, where 18 per cent and 14 per cent respectively of currently married couples were using condoms. Nationally, over the nineties, the extent of use of male/couple-dependent methods has remained the same. At the state level, all the southern states recorded a decline in the proportion of currently married couples using male/couple-dependent methods during the nineties (a decline ranging from 21 per cent to 46 per cent). Among the four major northern states, while Madhya Pradesh and Bihar recorded a decline, the proportion of couples using male methods increased in Rajasthan and Uttar Pradesh.

Contraceptive discontinuation and switching

As contraceptive use increases and becomes a more established behaviour, prevalence is no longer a sufficient marker of programme success (Jejeebhoy, 1990). Contraceptive continuation may become more important than acceptance in increasing contraceptive prevalence (Jain, 1989).

In India, as the vast majority (66 per cent) of ever users are sterilised, only a small proportion of ever users have the option of discontinuing use. Nationally, data from NFHS 2 show that one in ten currently married women who have ever used a contraceptive method (which translates into 29 per cent of ever users of reversible methods) had discontinued use at the time of the survey. The data also show that younger women (15-24-year-olds) were more likely to discontinue using contraceptives compared to older women. Younger women were also more likely to mention desire for a child but less likely to mention side effects as their main reason for discontinuation. However, younger women were no more likely than older women to discontinue use due to method failure or difficulty in accessing a suitable method. Notably, contraceptive discontinuation was comparatively higher in the northern and northeastern states, particularly the latter, than in the southern states. Moreover, women who discontinued using contraceptives in the northern and north-eastern states more frequently reported difficulty in accessing a method or inconvenience in using a method as reasons for discontinuation, compared with women in the southern states (IIPS and ORC Macro, 2000). Studies show higher discontinuation levels for oral contraceptive pills and condoms than IUDs (Gandotra and Das, 1996; Zhang, Tsui and Suchindran, 1999). The tendency to discontinue use seems to be more common in rural areas than in urban areas (Mari Bhat and Hasalkar, 1996).

Information on patterns of contraceptive switching is limited. An analysis of data on future use of contraception available from NFHS 2 sheds light on the intended pattern of switching among current discontinuers and indicates that one-third intend to use another method within 12 months from the time of the survey, another one-third intend to use a method some time later, and the rest do not intend to use any method at all. While nearly one-half (46 per cent) of the potential contraceptive switchers plan to use female sterilisation, one-fifth plan to switch to pills, one-tenth to condoms and another one-tenth to natural family planning. Among discontinuers who intend to switch to a method within 12 months, the choice tends to be more in favour of reversible methods (48 per cent for modern reversible methods, 10 per cent for natural family planning methods and 33 per cent for non-reversible methods). A prospective follow-up study of IUD users in Gujarat shows that approximately one-third of those who discontinued use after 12-18 months did not switch to any other method, one in ten switched to female sterilisation, one in twenty to natural methods, 3 per cent to oral pills and 3 per cent to condoms (Gandotra and Das, 1996).

Unmet need for contraception

Despite improved availability and access to contraceptive services, a substantial proportion of pregnancies (21 per cent of all pregnancies that resulted in live births nationally) were unplanned (mistimed or unwanted) (IIPS and ORC Macro, 2000). It is estimated that if all unwanted births could be eliminated, the total fertility rate would drop to the replacement level of fertility. Moreover, several studies report that the desire to limit family size and to space the next birth are the main reasons mentioned by the majority of abortion seekers (Ganatra, 2000), clearly highlighting that there is a substantial unmet need for contraception among women in India.

NFHS 2 reports that 16 per cent of currently married women have an unmet contraceptive need, which translates into one-fourth of women who wished to space or limit births (IIPS and ORC Macro, 2000). Based on the current population of 1,027 million, this implies that approximately 40 million married women have an unmet need (National Commission on Population, 2002). While the needs of the vast majority of women who wished to stop childbearing are being satisfied, the needs of women who wished to delay or space childbearing remain largely unsatisfied. For example, it is estimated that the needs of 86 per cent of women who wished to stop childbearing are addressed by the existing services, compared to the needs of 30 per cent of women who wished to delay their next pregnancy.

Young women are more likely to have an unmet need for contraception. According to NFHS 2 data, 25 per cent of young women, compared to 17 per cent of women aged 25-34 years and 7 per cent of women above 35 years, had an unmet need for contraception (IIPS and ORC Macro, 2000). When translated in terms of young women who wished to space or limit births, this implies that

Figure 1

Trends in unmet need for spacing and limiting

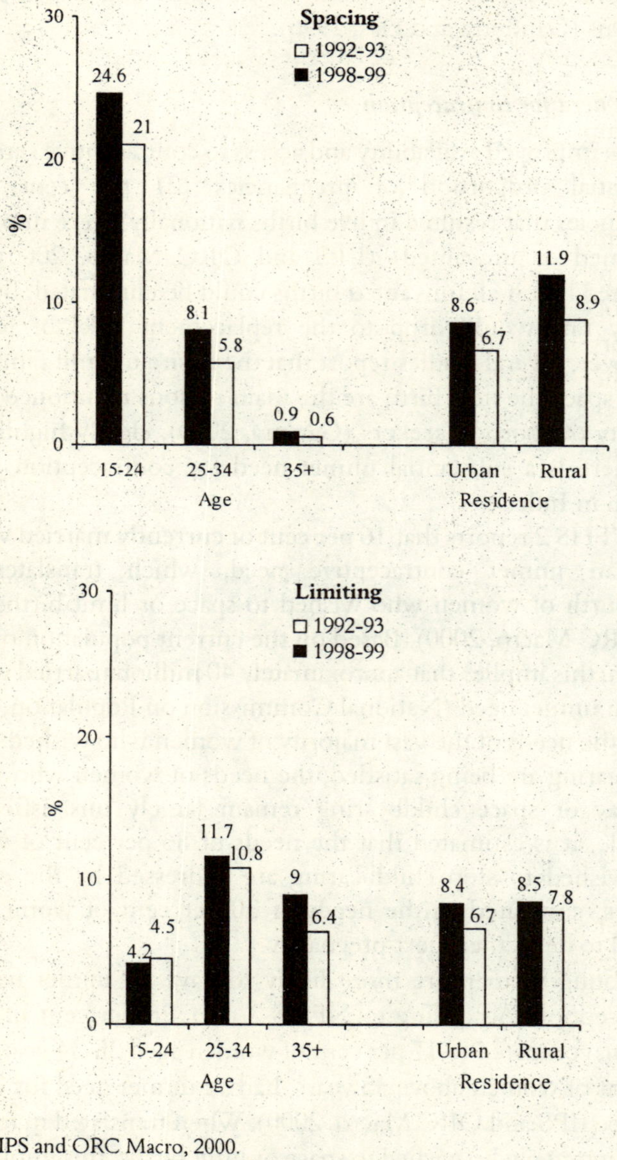

Source: IIPS and ORC Macro, 2000.

the existing service delivery system is addressing the contraceptive needs of only 44 per cent of young women. Among women who have not given birth, the contraceptive needs of only 25 per cent of women are satisfied (IIPS and ORC Macro, 2000). In addition to the strong programmatic emphasis on sterilisation until recently, this may be partly due to the neglect of young women by the programme that perceives a contraceptive need among young people only after they have completed their family formation. Evidence is emerging, however, that young couples, despite community norms that favour a first child soon after marriage, would prefer delaying the first birth until they have spent more time together getting to know each other better (Haberland, McGrory and Santhya, 2001).

There are pronounced regional differences in the proportion of women with an unmet need for contraception. NFHS 2 shows that the level of unmet need is higher in the northern and north-eastern states than in the southern states—19 per cent vs. 11 per cent. There are substantial differences in unmet need within each region as well. In the southern states, for example, 8 per cent of married women in Andhra Pradesh had an unmet need for contraception, compared to 17 per cent in Goa. Similarly, the level of unmet need in the northern states ranged from 7 per cent in Punjab to 25 per cent in Bihar and Uttar Pradesh, and in the north-eastern states from 16 per cent in Mizoram to 36 per cent in Meghalaya (IIPS and ORC Macro, 2000).

The proportion of women with an unmet need declined by 19 per cent during the six years between NFHS 1 and NFHS 2; the decline was more pronounced in the case of unmet need for spacing (by 25 per cent) than for limiting (12 per cent) (see Figure 1).

Barriers to meeting contraceptive needs

The family planning programme has been successful in improving contraceptive acceptance and reducing fertility rates but its achievements have been modest. While contextual and structural factors (high levels of illiteracy, poor access to sources of knowledge, poverty, gender and non-gender-based disparities) are partly responsible, the direction, emphasis and strategies followed hitherto in the family welfare programme have largely contributed to the limited success of the programme.

Limited knowledge

As is known, the small family norm is widely accepted (the mean ideal family size reported by young people currently is 2.5 children) and general awareness of contraception is universal (99 per cent of currently married women in the reproductive age group were aware of a contraceptive method). However, awareness of reversible (modern or natural) methods is relatively limited among both women and men. Nationally, for example, only 71 per cent of currently married women were aware of condoms (IIPS and ORC Macro, 2000). In some major states including Andhra Pradesh, Karnataka, Madhya Pradesh and Orissa, fewer than three in five currently married women were aware of condoms. Awareness of specific reversible methods that are suitable for young women was even more limited among young women compared to other women. For example, only three-fifths of married adolescents were aware of condoms, compared to nearly three-fourths of women between 20-34 years (Santhya and Jejeebhoy, 2003). Small-scale studies show that a substantial proportion of unmarried boys and girls also lack contraceptive knowledge (Bhende, 1994; Kumar et al., 2000b).

Inadequate knowledge of contraceptive methods, and incomplete or erroneous information about where to obtain methods and how to use them are the main reasons for not accepting family planning (Levine et al., 1992; Roy et al., 1991; Viswanathan, Godfrey and Yinger, 1998). Studies assessing correct, adequate and timely knowledge suggest that a small proportion have complete knowledge of various contraceptive methods (Balaiah et al., 1999; Rajaretnam and Deshpande, 1994; Sharma et al., 1997).

In many cases, men and women who were aware of contraceptive methods did not have timely knowledge. Studies show that had these couples had such knowledge during the initial years of their married life, they might have delayed the first pregnancy (Haberland, McGrory and Santhya, 2001; Levine et al., 1992; Santhya, McGrory and Haberland, 2001).

Gender inequalities and limited male involvement

Within the patriarchal set-up in India, women have relatively little power. The role of the husband has been noted in several studies of decision-making related to the use of contraception, especially during the early years of marriage (Acharya and Sureender, 1996; Barua and Kurz, 2001; Dharmalingam, 1995; Ghosh, 2001; Haberland, McGrory and Santhya, 2001; Jejeebhoy and Kulkarni, 1996; Ravindran, 1993). Most couples do not discuss with each other when to have their first child, birth spacing or contraception (Gupta, Jain and Sen, 2001; IIPS and ORC Macro, 2000; Khan and Patel, 1997). Nationally, for example, fewer than one in five currently married women reported discussing family planning with their husbands (IIPS and ORC Macro 2000). Studies also show that most men approve of contraception only after having a second or third child (Khan and Patel, 1997), and that husbands' approval of a particular method is critical (Parveen et al., 1995).

Though the need for promoting shared responsibility and the active involvement of men to improve reproductive health for all has been acknowledged, men's roles have not been properly defined in government programmes. There have been some programme efforts to promote the use of male methods such as vasectomy and condoms, and initiatives to re-popularise vasectomy, including information, education and communication (IEC) campaigns and training of surgeons in 'no-scalpel' vasectomy have been launched in several states (MOHFW, 1999). Though these efforts have proved to be successful in some districts in Andhra Pradesh, a similar change has not occurred in most other states (Planning Commission, 2002a).

Male health workers could play an important role in promoting male involvement in reproductive and child health. However, two-thirds of primary health centres in India do not have a male health worker (IIPS, 2001b). Moreover, the Reproductive and Child Health Programme document offers no clear guidelines on the role of male workers (Prakasamma, 1999a). The experience in Karnataka shows that male workers who traditionally focused on malaria and tuberculosis screening and follow-up view reproductive and child health as the domain of the female worker (Murthy et al., 2002).

Limited informed choice

The public sector essentially provides five contraceptive methods—two forms of tubectomy (laproscopy and minilap), vasectomy (including 'no-scalpel' vasectomy), IUDs (Copper T200), oral pills (combined) and condoms. Efforts to broaden the basket of choices have been under way including clinical trials to assess the safety and efficacy of available methods such as estrogen-progestogen combination injectables, vaginal rings and long-acting IUDs, and the development of new methods of male and female fertility regulation (Puri, 1998). As part of expanding contraceptive choice, the government has introduced emergency contraceptive pills in the Reproductive and Child Health Programme (MOHFW, 2002a). However, most women and men, particularly those who rely on the public sector (76 per cent of current users of modern methods rely on the public sector, IIPS and ORC Macro, 2000), do not have access to a wide choice of contraceptives. Methods that are perceived as less effective including pessaries, spermicides, diaphragms, or are controversial including injectables and implants are dropped from the public programme, not introduced or given low priority by health workers. The recently introduced emergency contraceptive pills are currently available through medical officers only at the district and sub-district level (Mallik, 2003).

Not only is access to a wider choice of methods limited, but providers also often do not assist women and men to exercise their right to contraceptive choice by offering them complete and accurate information on the variety of methods available. Nationally, for example, only 15 per cent of users of modern contraceptive methods who were motivated by a health worker from the public or private sector were informed of at least one alternative method (IIPS and ORC Macro, 2000). Private and NGO sector health workers were more likely to inform clients of alternative methods than were public sector health workers (28 per cent vs. 19 per cent) (IIPS and ORC Macro, 2000). Several small-scale studies report that most providers have a distinct bias towards sterilisation and only a minority of clients were informed of reversible methods (Barge and Ramachandar, 1999; ICMR, 1991; Khan, Patel and Chandrasekhar 1993; Khan, Gupta and Patel, 1999; Khan, Patel and Gupta, 1999; Murthy, 1999; Ravindran, 1999; Roy and Verma, 1999; Verma and Roy, 1999; Visaria, 1999a; 2000).

In spite of evidence that pre-acceptance counselling improves contraceptive continuation (ICMR Task Force on IUD and Hormonal Contraceptives, 1994; Prabhavati and Sheshadri, 1988), counselling of clients on how the method works, what the expected side effects are and how to manage the side effects is typically lacking or limited in the family welfare programme. Nationally, data from NFHS 2 indicate that only 22 per cent of users of any modern method were informed of its possible side effects at the time of accepting the method (IIPS and ORC Macro, 2000). Similarly, data from the Reproductive and Child Health Survey report that only one-third of sterilisation users (35 per cent), less than one-half of IUD users (46 per cent) and less than one-fourth of pill users (23 per cent) were informed of side effects before accepting the method (IIPS, 2001a).

Research on users' perspectives/client acceptability of methods is limited, but available evidence suggests that many of these methods are acceptable to women in rural and urban areas (Rajgopal et al., 1989; Ravindran, 1995a). Evidence is emerging that if provided with detailed information on all available contraceptive methods, women do make an informed choice overriding the provider's bias. For example, in a study where potential clients were provided with detailed information on various methods such as IUDs, oral pills, condoms, sterilisation and Norplant, the majority (80 per cent) opted for reversible methods, irrespective of their literacy status, and only 17 per cent accepted sterilisation (Baveja et al., 2000).

Limited access and availability of services

Over the decades, there has been considerable expansion and strengthening of the health care infrastructure, and family welfare services are now an integral part of services provided by primary, secondary and tertiary care institutions across the country. Currently, approximately 137,271 subcentres (1/4,579 population) and 22,975 primary health centres (1/27,364 population) in the rural areas, and 871 health posts and 1,083 family welfare centres in urban areas provide family planning services at the grassroots level (Planning Commission, 2002a). Access to contraceptive methods has increased significantly, and only a negligible minority of women (4 per cent as per NFHS 2 data, IIPS and ORC Macro, 2000) perceive availability, accessibility or cost as major impediments to using contraception. Yet, in practice, access to and availability of services are significant issues of concern.

Where workers are available, they are generally poorly trained and have little knowledge of the methods they are to provide (Foo and Koenig, 2000; Jejeebhoy and Kulkarni, 1996). A facility survey observes that only 16 per cent of primary health centres have physicians trained in conducting sterilisation, and only two-thirds have at least one paramedical staff trained in IUD insertion (IIPS, 2001b). While female health workers in many studies reported that they had received training in IUD insertion, the majority did not feel confident about actually inserting an IUD in field settings or showed little awareness of the precautions to be taken (Visaria, 2000). The Reproductive and Child Health Programme has laid greater emphasis on skill upgradation and gender sensitisation training, and a nation-wide reproductive and child health training programme has been launched to upgrade the skills of health providers and managers to deliver the package of reproductive and child health services. A mid-term review of the reproductive and child health training programme has noted that the training focuses more on the technical aspects of service delivery and gives little importance to areas such as client needs and quality of services (Mavalankar, 2002b).

Health and family planning workers are required to regularly visit households in their assigned areas to provide information related to health and family planning, counsel and motivate women to adopt appropriate health and family planning practices, and deliver other related services. However, data from NFHS 2 indicate that only 13 per cent of women had received a home visit from a health and family planning worker during the 12 months preceding the survey and only 11 per cent of women who were visited at home reported that they received family planning services. Women without any children were least likely to receive a home visit (IIPS and ORC Macro, 2000). State-level data show that less than 2 per cent of women in many states including Arunachal Pradesh, Delhi, Haryana, Jammu and Kashmir, Nagaland and Punjab received a home visit from a health and family planning worker in the 12 months preceding the survey. In only four states—Gujarat, Mizoram, Tamil Nadu and Maharashtra—did at least a quarter of women receive such visits. Several small-scale studies also reveal significant shortcomings in the frequency and regularity of outreach services, the time devoted by workers to such activities and the length of time spent with clients (Foo and Koenig, 2000). Additionally, outreach services were reported to be almost non-existent in remote and tribal areas (Murthy, 1999). Moreover, health workers at the community level were often looked upon with distrust, and identified as interested only in recruiting 'cases' for family planning (Jejeebhoy and Kulkarni, 1996; Ravindran, 1993). The introduction of the Target-free Approach/Community Needs Assessment Approach, however, has reportedly enabled front-line health workers to gain a more positive image in their communities (Murthy et al., 2002; Sathyanarayana and Kar, 2001; Sen, Gurumurthy and Sudarshan, 1999).

The Reproductive and Child Health Programme recommends that women who do not deliver in institutions should receive three postpartum visits during which they are to be provided with advice on family planning. Data from NFHS 2 show not only that postpartum check-ups are almost non-existent but also that family planning is given the lowest priority among the various components of postpartum care (IIPS and ORC Macro, 2000). Nationally, fewer than one in five non-institutional births were followed by a postpartum check-up. Among those who received a postpartum check-up, only 27 per cent of mothers received advice on family planning, compared to 43 per cent receiving advice on breastfeeding and 46 per cent receiving advice on baby care. Adolescent mothers and women delivering for the first time were less likely than older women to receive advice on family planning. Notably, mothers received advice on family planning during postpartum check-ups for only 14 per cent of first births, although these women are more likely to need advice on birth spacing and contraception. Clearly health workers and other providers tend to overlook adolescent and young women until they are further advanced in their reproductive careers.

Stock-outs and erratic supplies of reversible contraceptives make it unrealistic to expect providers to offer clients a choice of methods. A survey reports that only 56-61 per cent of primary health centres had some stocks of condoms, IUDs and oral pills on the day of the survey. The situation was worse in states like Bihar, Orissa and Uttar Pradesh where fewer than one-fifth of the primary health centres had some stocks of these methods (IIPS, 2001b).

Many new initiatives, the restructuring of existing measures, particularly those undertaken by NGOs, and some experiments with public-private partnerships have been successful in improving access to and availability of contraceptive and other reproductive health services. The social marketing and social franchising of selected reproductive health services by Janani, a registered society in Bihar (Gopalakrishnan et al., 2002), and the experience of the Innovations in Family Planning Services project in Uttar Pradesh (Levitt-Dayal, 2002) are examples of such success.

Poor quality of services

It is now widely acknowledged that the quality of family planning services is generally poor. Little consideration is given to interpersonal interactions (Gupta, 1993; Levine et al., 1992; Mavalankar and Sharma, 1999; Ramachandar and Barge, 1999; Ravindran, 1999; Ramanathan, Dilip and Padmadas, 1995). Service providers tend to be insensitive and disregard women's need for privacy. Pre-acceptance counselling or check-ups are limited, and little attention is paid to post-acceptance follow-up services. Nationally, for example, data from NFHS 2 show that three in four sterilisation users and two in five users of other modern methods received follow-up services (IIPS and ORC Macro, 2000). The data also show that although the quality of family planning services is far from satisfactory in all the states, the quality of services is poorer in states such as Arunachal Pradesh, Orissa, Uttar Pradesh and West Bengal.

Changing policy and programme environment

The family planning programme in India, launched in 1951, has evolved through a number of stages and has changed its direction, emphasis and strategies. The 1990s particularly witnessed dramatic changes in the family welfare policy and programme. With the 72nd and 73rd Constitutional amendments and the passing of the Panchayati Raj and Nagar Palika Acts in 1992, the family planning programme was legally brought in the domain of panchayati raj institutions. In 1996, the target-oriented approach was replaced with the Target-free Approach, where health workers' case loads would be determined by needs identified at the community level rather than set at the central or state level. In 1997, to direct the programme more towards clients' needs, the Target-free Approach was recast as the Community Needs Assessment Approach, and decentralised participatory planning was brought in place. In the same year, the Reproductive and Child Health Programme was launched. The Reproductive and Child Health Programme espouses the principles of client satisfaction and high quality in delivering comprehensive and integrated health services.

The National Population Policy, adopted in February 2000, further legitimised the shift towards incorporating quality of care within public sector services. The National Population Policy provides a policy framework for achieving the twin objectives of population stabilisation and promoting reproductive health within the wider context of sustainable development. The immediate objective of the policy is to address the unmet need for contraception and to provide integrated service delivery for basic reproductive and child health care. In the medium term, the policy seeks to achieve the goal of bringing the total fertility rates to replacement level by 2010 through vigorous implementation of inter-sectoral operational strategies (MOHFW, 2000). The National Population Policy affirms the government's commitment to the provision of quality services, information and counselling, and expanding contraceptive method choices in order to enable people to make voluntary and informed choices.

The strategies delineated in the new policies are currently under way with varying intensity and clarity in different parts of the country. It is too early to make definitive assessments about the impact of the new initiatives. However, early assessments suggest that although a decentralised, participative planning process through community needs assessment has begun, it requires considerable refinement to become effectively functional (Narayana and Sangawan, 2001). Uncertain of the consequences of the new approach, many states continue to impose targets, setting local goals based on the previous year's centrally assigned targets (Visaria, Jejeebhoy and Merrick, 1999). Women's involvement in the process of decentralised decision-making at the grassroots has yet to be operationalised. In many states, the involvement of the community and other stakeholders, including panchayati raj institutions, in community needs assessment is reported to be minimal (Planning Commission, 2002a; World Bank, 2000).

The way forward

Though the family planning programme has experienced significant growth and expansion over the past half century, pregnancies continue to be unplanned and the unmet need for contraception remains substantially high. Important sub-groups, such as adolescents, are neglected or under-served, the vast majority of contraceptive users are sterilised, contraceptive choice is conspicuous by its absence and quality of care is limited within the programme.

The 1990s witnessed a growing recognition of the challenges faced by the programme that led to the development of several new policy initiatives. The programme focus has shifted from vertical family planning services towards the provision of comprehensive integrated reproductive health care. Early assessment of the impact of the new policy and programme initiatives suggests some improvements in overall indicators such as contraceptive prevalence rates and the magnitude of unmet need for contraception. However, underlying issues including limited contraceptive choice, poor quality of services, restricted access, gender inequalities and lack of male involvement continue to plague the programme. Mechanisms to address these issues remain elusive and the strategies outlined in policies to address these core issues remain poorly implemented.

Programme recommendations

- An expanded reproductive health programme must address men both in terms of their own health needs and in terms of their shared responsibility as partners, husbands and fathers and should not be limited to promoting the use of male contraceptive methods. The role of male health workers who could play an active role in promoting male involvement also needs to be clearly defined.

- The contraceptive needs of sexually active young people remain largely unmet. Young people, married as well as unmarried, need accurate, user-friendly information and services. Multiple entry points (education, work, sports, or other social activities) and settings (home, community, workplace, school or clinic) must be used to enhance access to information and services.
- Provider bias continues to restrict the rights of women and men in exercising contraceptive choice. The providers need to be oriented about the clients' rights to exercise choice. Additionally, a variety of providers, including traditional medical practitioners, should be trained and engaged to promote detailed information on various contraceptive methods.
- Given that women, especially young women, are powerless and voiceless in sexual and reproductive matters, multi-sectoral activities to enhance women's status are much needed. Since reproductive decision-making is often beyond the control of young women and their husbands, engaging other gatekeepers including senior men and women in the family and influential people in the community is crucial.
- IEC efforts to enable clients to exercise informed contraceptive choice have been increased, but inadequate collaboration between the health sector, IEC units and other stakeholders is reportedly rendering these efforts ineffective. Hence, inter-sectoral coordination needs to be vigorously promoted.
- The involvement of the community in planning and monitoring remains minimal. Concerted efforts to promote community participation are needed.
- As reflected throughout in this review, there are substantial state-level variations in contraceptive prevalence, the method-mix commonly used, the extent of unmet need, the level of awareness of reversible methods, and the quality of

services. This clearly highlights the importance of state-specific interventions to improve family planning services.

Research recommendations

- Research on the attitude and practice of men regarding fertility regulation, and the factors inhibiting their role and participation in reproductive health could help improve and modify the delivery system. Research is also required to determine men's needs for services and information in specific communities. Operations research is required to assess how educational campaigns could be made effective to promote shared responsibilities. As methods of fertility regulation available to men are limited, priority should be given to developing male methods of family planning.
- Gaining a better understanding of how women and men make choices and negotiate trade-offs among methods could provide useful insights for policy makers, programme managers as well as clients themselves. Future research should explore the context in which women and men exercise choice, including the power dynamics of relationships, and the interface between clients and the service system.
- Additional research is required to understand why women discontinue use, and whether efforts to provide detailed information under the new programmes have improved contraceptive continuation rates. Similarly, explorations into whether the new rhetoric on quality of care has been translated into reality and impacted contraceptive use dynamics are critically needed.
- Apart from data from Reproductive and Child Health Survey-2 currently under way and a few small-scale studies, detailed and in-depth insights into the impact of new initiatives are scarce. Qualitative studies are needed to assess the perspectives of primary and secondary stakeholders regarding the changes in the programme.

Maternal Health and Pregnancy-related Care

Shireen J. Jejeebhoy and Leila Caleb Varkey

Each year, in India, roughly 30 million women experience pregnancy and 27 million have a live birth (MOHFW, 2003c). Of these, over 100,000 maternal deaths and one million newborn deaths occur annually. Millions more suffer pregnancy related ill health. Although pregnancy-related mortality and morbidity continue to take a huge toll on the lives of women and newborns, and despite a series of programmatic initiatives, there is little evidence that maternity has become significantly safer over the last 20 years. On the positive side, the Tenth Plan and the Reproductive and Child Health Programme have set the country on an ambitious course towards improving pregnancy-related health by the year 2007.

Maternal and neonatal mortality: Trends, causes and correlates

Trends

It is generally accepted that maternal mortality is difficult to measure and even more difficult to track over time. Direct and indirect estimates agree, however, that maternal mortality remains unacceptably high in India. For example, direct measures obtained from NFHS 1 and 2 (covering the period 1992-93 and 1998-99 respectively, available only at the national level) suggest a ratio of 424 per 100,000 births and 540 per 100,000 live births in the two years preceding NFHS 1 and NFHS 2 respectively (IIPS, 1995; IIPS and ORC Macro, 2000). Likewise, data from the Sample Registration System report maternal mortality ratios of 437 and 408 per 100,000 live births in 1993 and 1998, respectively (RGI, 1999-2000; 2000). Sampling errors are large and fail to establish statistically that there has been any change over the six-year period. Indirect estimates hint however of a steady decline in maternal mortality ratios: from 580 per 100,000 live births in 1982-86 to 519 in 1987-1991 to 440 by 1992-96 (Mari Bhat, 2002; Mari Bhat, Navaneetham and Iruyada Rajan, 1995; see Figure 2).

Figure 2

Trends in Estimated Maternal Mortality Ratios, India, 1955-95

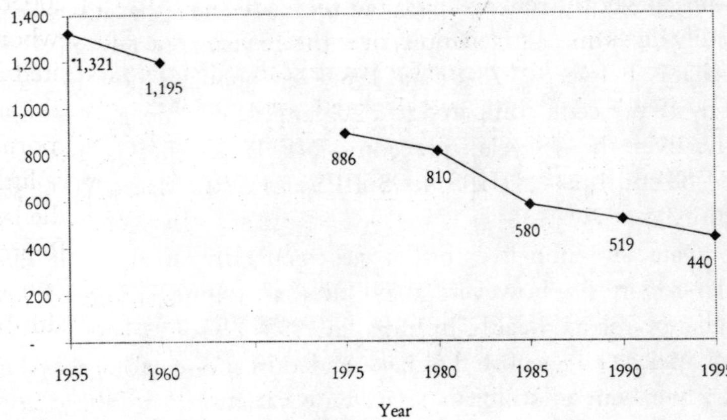

Source: Mari Bhat, 2002.

The neonatal mortality rate currently stands at 43.4 per 1,000 live births (for the five years preceding NFHS 2, 1998-99) (IIPS and ORC Macro, 2000). Like maternal mortality ratios, mortality

Figure 3

Neonatal Mortality Rates for Five-Year Periods (approx. 1978-98)

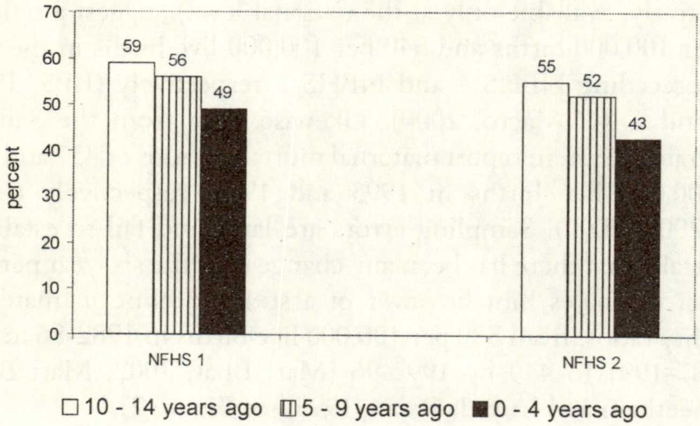

Source: IIPS 1995; IIPS and ORC Macro, 2000.

among newborns remains high but there are signs that it has been steadily declining. For example, over the 15 years preceding NFHS 1—that is, between 1978-82 and 1988-92—neonatal mortality rates fell by 18 per cent, compared to a 20 per cent decline, correspondingly, over the 15 years preceding NFHS 2—that is, between 1984-88 and 1994-98 (IIPS, 1995; IIPS and ORC Macro, 2000; see Figure 3).

Data on non-live births are generally inadequate and under-reported, however they are a telling indicator of pregnancy-related health. In India, in 1998-99, some 4 per cent of pregnancies were reported to have ended in spontaneous abortion and 2 per cent in stillbirth. State-wise variation for stillbirths is narrow, varying from 1.1 per cent in Goa to 3.3 per cent in Meghalaya (IIPS and ORC Macro, 2000).

Over the course of the 1990s, maternal mortality (indirect estimates) fell by roughly 15 per cent and neonatal mortality by 11 per cent (Mari Bhat, 2002; IIPS and ORC Macro, 2000). By 2007, the country aims to achieve a maternal mortality ratio of 200 per

100,000 live births and a neonatal mortality rate of 26 per 1,000 live births (see Table 2) (MOHFW, 2000; Planning Commission, 2002b). Indeed, the goal is to achieve—between the late 1990s and 2007, that is, in less than a decade—a virtual halving of the maternal mortality ratio and a 40 per cent decline in the neonatal mortality rate.

Table 2

The maternal and neonatal mortality scenario and goals for 2007

	Maternal mortality ratio		*Neonatal Mortality Rate***
	*Indirect**	*NFHS***	
Early 1990s	519	424	48.6
Late 1990s	440	540	43.4
Goal for 2007#	200		26.0

Source: * Mari Bhat, 2002; **IIPS and ORC Macro, 2000; # Planning Commission, 2002b.

State-wise variation

Regional disparities in maternal and neonatal mortality are wide. Maternal mortality is so low in such states as Kerala and Punjab that indirect estimates for these states could not be attempted; in contrast in as many as 10 of the 15 major states (Assam, Bihar, Gujarat, Haryana, Karnataka, Madhya Pradesh, Orissa, Rajasthan, Uttar Pradesh and West Bengal) ratios exceed 400 per 100,000 live births, and in three states (Assam, Madhya Pradesh and Uttar Pradesh) are as high as 700 or more (Mari Bhat, 2002). Direct evidence from NFHS suggests, likewise, considerable rural-urban variation: as expected, the rural maternal mortality ratio was considerably higher than the urban in both the early and late 1990s: 434 as compared to 385 in NFHS 1 and 619 and 267, respectively in NFHS 2 (note that these are affected by large confidence intervals and sampling errors; IIPS, 1995; IIPS and ORC Macro, 2000).

State-wise variation is evident in the case of neonatal mortality as well. While Kerala reports a neonatal mortality rate (for the five-year period preceding NFHS 2) of 13.8, some five major states report neonatal mortality rates of over 45 per 1,000 births (Bihar including Jharkhand, Madhya Pradesh including Chhattisgarh, Orissa, Rajasthan and Uttar Pradesh including Uttaranchal)—notably those in the northern region and classified, on the basis of their socio-demographic indicators, as empowered action group (EAG) states requiring concerted programmatic effort.

Causes of death

Common causes of maternal death are those seen in most developing country settings and are largely preventable. Estimates derived from data on maternal deaths, collected through the Sample Registration System, may not be entirely accurate because of small sample sizes and difficulties in ascertaining cause of death from household inquiries. However, they do provide a useful picture of the causes of death (RGI, 2000). Data on the causes of death were collected through post-death verbal autopsies conducted by non-medical field investigators. Haemorrhage and sepsis were the leading causes of maternal death even as recently as 1998 (30 per cent and 16 per cent of all maternal deaths respectively; see Table 3) (RGI, 2000). Other identifiable causes of death during pregnancy, childbirth and the postpartum period were obstructed labour, toxaemia and unsafe abortion. In addition, some 25 per cent of maternal deaths were attributed to indirect causes. Leading among these was reportedly anaemia (19 per cent); given that causes of death were assessed by non-medical persons through verbal autopsies, we assume that such causes as "weakness" without indications of bleeding, swelling or fever may have been reported as anaemia (see also Bhatia, 1993; Ganatra, Coyaji and Rao, 1998). Likewise, a study comparing pregnancy-related complications among women who died (through verbal autopsies) and those who survived in three states (Andhra Pradesh, Madhya Pradesh and Orissa) confirms that of the 170 deaths studied, leading causes were sepsis ("high fever"), obstructed labour and excessive bleeding (Murthy and Barua, 2001).

Table 3

Causes of maternal death, 1998 (%)

Cause	%
Direct causes	
Haemorrhage	29.6
Puerperal sepsis	16.1
Obstructed labour	9.5
Abortion	8.9
Toxaemia	8.3
Indirect causes	
Anaemia	19.0
Tuberculosis	4.6
Malaria	1.4
Viral hepatitis	0.4

Source: RGI, 2000.

Deaths of newborns during the first week or month of life are largely the result of inadequate or inappropriate care during pregnancy, childbirth or the first critical hours after birth. Indeed, neonatal mortality (largely dependent on maternal and pregnancy-related health) continues to account for almost two-thirds of all infant deaths, and has been declining at a somewhat slower pace than post-neonatal mortality (largely dependent on exogenous factors). For example, over the period 1992-93 to 1998-99, the neonatal mortality rate (for the five years preceding the NFHS survey) declined by 10.7 per cent while the post-neonatal mortality rate recorded a corresponding decline of 19 per cent (IIPS, 1995; IIPS and ORC Macro, 2000).

Major causes of neonatal mortality include neonatal infections (tetanus, sepsis, meningitis, pneumonia and congenital syphilis), birth asphyxia and trauma, pre-term birth and/or low birth weight, and other causes, including congenital anomalies, accounting for some 52 per cent, 20 per cent, 15 per cent and 13 per cent of all deaths nationally (Planning Commission, 2002b).

Recent investigations using verbal autopsy highlight the extent to which prematurity, low birth weight, birth asphyxia and neonatal sepsis were leading causes of death of neonates (Gupta and Keyl, 1998; Kapoor et al., 1996; Shrivastava, Kumar and Ojha, 2001).

Correlates

Maternal and neonatal mortality are undoubtedly influenced by such contextual factors as poverty, access to health care and overall levels of development. Available evidence reiterates the strong association between such socio-demographic factors as women's education, age and parity and maternal and neonatal mortality.

Education and standard of living

Indirect estimates suggest for example that maternal mortality among women with a middle school or higher education is lower than those who are uneducated (Mari Bhat, 2002). Likewise, neonatal mortality for the 10-year period preceding NFHS 2 was 55.3 among illiterate mothers compared to 24.3 among those with a high school or better education, and 55.8 compared to 30.9 per 1,000 live births among those with low and high standards of living, respectively (IIPS and ORC Macro, 2000). Findings of an in-depth case study of pregnancy-related experiences in three states (Andhra Pradesh, Madhya Pradesh and Orissa) confirm likewise that women who experienced maternal death were more likely to be poorly educated and to live in kuccha homes than those who survived (Murthy and Barua, 2001).

Age

Early onset of marriage and childbearing in India continues to have disturbing consequences for maternal health. The median age at first cohabitation with husband is 17 years among women aged 25-49 (IIPS and ORC Macro, 2000), and cultural pressures make it imperative for a women's security in her marital home for her to conceive as soon as possible after marriage. The median age at first birth is, therefore, early—19.4 years among women aged 25-49. In other words, half of all women had already experienced pregnancy and childbearing by the time they were 19, often before full physical maturity is attained. As a result of the combined effects of shorter average maternal height, competition for nutrients between mother's growth needs and the growth needs of her foetus, and poorer placental functions of adolescent mothers, the pregnant adolescent is particularly at risk (Leslie, 1991). Community and facility level data have reiterated that adolescents are more likely to experience maternal death than adult women. For example, a national study conducted by ICMR of 43,550 women in 10 facilities reports that maternal mortality among adolescents (aged under 20) was 645/100,000 live births, compared to 342/100,000 among women aged 20-34 years (Krishna, 1995).

While data on the link between age and maternal mortality are sparse, national-level data suggest that adolescent mothers are considerably more likely than mothers aged 20-29 to experience adverse pregnancy outcomes, notably higher neonatal mortality (63 and 41 respectively) (IIPS and ORC Macro, 2000). Corresponding disparities in post-neonatal deaths are in comparison mild (30 and 23). Likewise, hospital-based and community-level studies report that compared to women aged 20-29, adolescents experienced higher rates of perinatal mortality, spontaneous abortion and stillbirth (Hirve and Ganatra, 1994; Khandait et al., 2000; Pachauri and Jamshedji, 1983; Verma and Das, 1997).

Parity and previous birth intervals

Parity has a similar effect. Mortality is especially high among nulliparous women, declines sharply among women at parities 1-3, and rises sharply among higher parity women. The link to previous birth intervals is evident at the national level: neonatal mortality rates fell from 72 per 1,000 live births among women with a birth interval of 24 months or less to 24 among those with an interval of 48 months or more (IIPS and ORC Macro, 2000).

Maternal and neonatal morbidity: Levels and correlates

Levels

Community-level studies of maternal and neonatal morbidity are rare and most focus on a limited geographical area. The recent exception is the NFHS which not only obtained self-reported data of health problems during pregnancy and complications during the postpartum stage experienced by women who gave birth during the three years preceding the survey but also assessed levels of anaemia experienced by all women. However, findings must be interpreted cautiously as self-reported morbidity experiences may be influenced by recall problems (if information is obtained retrospectively) or by women's tendency to consider many conditions as normal events in a woman's life.

Studies uniformly raise concern about significant levels of maternal and neonatal morbidity. At the national level, findings suggest that almost half of all women were anaemic (48 per cent) and some 17 per cent suffered moderate or severe anaemia. Considerable state-wise variation is evident, ranging from 3.2 in Kerala to 15-20 per cent in the EAG states. Self-reported health problems during pregnancy are clearly exacerbated by already compromised levels of anaemia: excessive fatigue and anaemia (reported by 43 and 27 per cent respectively) were leading morbidities reported by recently pregnant women. In addition, women reported swelling of the legs, body or face (26 per cent), blurred vision (22 per cent) and convulsions not from fever (14 per cent). During the postpartum stage, 11 per cent of women experienced massive vaginal bleeding and 13 per cent experienced very high fever (IIPS and ORC Macro, 2000).

Following the pioneering community-based study highlighting significant pregnancy-related morbidity in rural Rajasthan (Datta et al., 1980), a number of recent studies have explored maternal morbidity in greater depth and shed more light on pregnancy and childbirth related morbidity patterns. For example, in rural Karnataka, as many as 41 per cent of all women reported at least one morbid condition associated with their last pregnancy: 18 per cent reported a morbidity in the antenatal period; another 18 per cent at delivery; and 23 per cent in the postpartum period. As many as 10 per cent of all women experienced a potentially life threatening morbidity in the antenatal period (swelling, fits and convulsions, hypertension, bleeding, high fever), 8 per cent during delivery (long labour, excessive bleeding, loss of consciousness, ruptured uterus, torn vagina or cervix, convulsions), and 11 per cent during the postpartum period (excessive bleeding, loss of consciousness, convulsions) (Bhatia and Cleland, 1996). In Tamil Nadu and Pondicherry, 45 per cent reported a serious or life-threatening morbidity: 25 per cent in the antenatal stage, 15 per cent in the intra-partum stage and 19 per cent in the postpartum stage (Srinivasa et al., 1997). Studies of pregnant women in the slums of Delhi and rural Karnataka similarly suggest considerable morbidity (Ganapathy, Ramakrishna and Matthews, 2000; Mayank et al., 2001).

Malnutrition and anaemia, both in adolescence and during pregnancy, are important precursors of complications during pregnancy, childbirth and thereafter, as well as perinatal and neonatal mortality and low birth weight. At the national level, as reported above, anaemia is widespread. Particularly affected are adolescents, namely, those who have or are about to experience pregnancy, among whom some 20 per cent are moderately or severely anaemic (IIPS and ORC Macro, 2000). Numerous studies confirm the relatively poor health and nutritional status of women, and wide-ranging gender disparities in feeding practices and prompt access to health care from an early age (Das Gupta, 1987; Khan et al., 1988; Srikantia, 1989). During pregnancy, malnourishment can increase. A recent study of pregnant women in Delhi slums reports that 45 per cent of pregnant women were malnourished, that is their caloric intake was less than 60 per cent of the recommended dietary allowance during pregnancy, and 80 per cent consumed less than the recommended daily amount; 40 per cent weighed less than 45 kg and 7 per cent were less than 145 cm in height (Bhandari and Mayank, 1999); two-thirds were anaemic and 12 per cent were severely anaemic (Mayank et al., 2001). A facility-based study concludes that highly anaemic women (Hb<8.9g per cent) were over four times as likely as those with higher haemoglobin levels (>11g per cent) to experience prolonged labour and abnormal deliveries (Malhotra et al., 2002).

Other pregnancy-related morbidities are also becoming increasingly apparent. Postnatal depression is observed. A prospective study in Goa of pregnant women followed up to six months postpartum noted depressive disorders among 23 per cent at 6-8 weeks following delivery and for more than half of these, symptoms persisted up to six months postpartum (Patel, Rodrigues and DeSouza, 2002).

An indicator of risk during pregnancy is the observation of HIV among pregnant women. Based on an analysis of 1999 sentinel surveillance data collected from 180 sites, the positivity rate among 16,661 pregnant women was 0.3 per cent, with the largest numbers in the age group 20-24 years. Current HIV prevalence in the antenatal population varies across states, from a low of 0 per cent to a high of 1.8 per cent. States such as Andhra Pradesh, Goa, Karnataka, Maharashtra, Manipur, Mizoram, Nagaland and Tamil Nadu report rates of 1 per cent or higher (NACO, 2003a; PFI and PRB, 2003). The presence of HIV seriously influences pregnancy and maternal and newborn health. For example, findings from facility-based studies in Manipur suggest that HIV has a significantly adverse effect upon maternal survival time and infant mortality as well as miscarriage, pre-term delivery and low birth weight (Kumar, Rizk and Khurranna, 1997; Kumar, Uduman and Khurranna, 1995).

There appears to be a disturbing trend towards caesarean section delivery in India. Although caesarean section rates nationally are not high—7 per cent of recently delivered women reported caesarean deliveries in 1998-99—analysis of NFHS 2 data suggests considerable rural-urban disparity (5 per cent and 15 per cent respectively) (IIPS and ORC Macro, 2000). Moreover, there is considerable state-wise variation: while rates are below 10 per cent in most states, caesarean section deliveries are particularly high in such high literacy states as Goa and Kerala (20 per cent and 29 per cent respectively) (IIPS and ORC Macro, 2000). There is also a suggestion that caesarean section deliveries may be increasing over time. A review of births in a hospital setting in Mumbai from 1957 to 1998 suggests that the proportion of caesarean deliveries increased from 1.9 per cent to 16 per cent in this period; after a threshold of 10 per cent was achieved, further increases in percentages delivered by caesarean section had no influence on improvement in perinatal mortality—on the contrary the more liberal use of caesarean deliveries may have increased perinatal mortality rates among those so delivered (Mehta et al., 2001). Findings also suggest, moreover, a strong association between private sector deliveries and caesarean section rates in all states; in Andhra Pradesh, Bihar, Gujarat, Karnataka, Punjab, Tamil Nadu and Uttar Pradesh, particularly, the risk of undergoing a caesarean section was four or more times higher in private facilities than in public sector facilities (Mishra and Ramanathan, 2002; Sreevidya and Sathiyasekaran, 2003). Such findings suggest the possible misuse of available technologies particularly in large urban centres with high proportions delivering in private facilities (Mishra and Ramanathan, 2002).

Conditions such as prolapse and fistulae are infrequently reported in studies of morbidity among recently delivered women, as these are longer-term sequalae of pregnancy. A study in south India that assessed long-term morbidity following delivery found that among 3,844 women who delivered up to 24 months prior to the study, 3 per cent experienced uterine prolapse and urinary incontinence and two women reported rectovaginal fistulae (Srinivasa et al., 1997). A synthesis of six community-based studies of gynaecological morbidity in India reports prolapse among 1 to 7 per cent of all women surveyed (Koenig et al., 1998).

Correlates

While the socio-demographic correlates of maternal and neonatal morbidity are not as well studied as the correlates of mortality, available evidence generally supports a strong association. With regard to age-specific differences in morbidity, for example, NFHS 1 reveals that adolescents were more likely to report morbidity than older women (IIPS, 1995). Likewise, facility-based studies in Mumbai and rural West Bengal report that compared to women aged 20-29, adolescents experienced more problems in the antenatal and intra-natal periods and more anaemia, pregnancy-induced hypertension and pre-term labour (Pachauri and Jamshedji, 1983; Verma and Das, 1997). A community-based study in rural Karnataka also observes significantly higher morbidity in the antenatal, natal and postpartum stages among nulliparous women than either women at parity 1-3 or 4 and more (Bhatia and Cleland, 1996). However, findings from the recent NFHS fail to establish these associations.

Studies in rural West Bengal and Maharashtra report, similarly, that teenage women were more likely to deliver pre-term and low birth weight babies compared to older women (Hirve and Ganatra, 1994; Verma and Das, 1997). Another study notes that even when exposed to identical levels of antenatal care and immunisation, and despite virtually identical levels of weight and haemoglobin at 20 weeks of pregnancy, adolescent mothers experienced poorer outcomes than adult mothers (Aras et al., 1989).

Pregnancy-related care

The links between pregnancy-related care and maternal mortality are well recognised, and over the last decade national programmes and Plans have stressed the need for universal screening of pregnant women and operationalising essential and emergency obstetric care. Goals set in the Tenth Plan advocate an ambitious agenda to make pregnancy safe, including the achievement of skilled attendance at 80 per cent of all deliveries by 2007, institutional deliveries for 65 per cent of all births, at least three antenatal check-ups for 90 per cent of pregnant women and universal achievement of complete immunisation for pregnant women (see Table 4).

Table 4
Pregnancy-related care: The current situation and goals for 2007 (%)

	1992-93	*1998-99*	*Goals for 2007*
Antenatal Care			
Women receiving no antenatal check-up	36.8	34.6	—
Women who received all recommended types of antenatal care	NA	20.0	—
Pregnant women receiving at least three antenatal check-ups	26.9*	43.8	90
Pregnant women receiving two or more doses of tetanus-toxoid	53.8	66.8	100
Intrapartum Care			
Women who delivered in a health facility/institution	25.5	33.6	65
Women attended by trained health personnel	34.2	42.3	80
Postpartum Care			
Women who received a postpartum check-up within 2 months of birth **	NA	16.5	—
Women who received a postpartum check-up within 2 days of birth **	NA	2.3	—

Source: IIPS, 1995; IIPS and ORC Macro, 2000; Planning Commission, 2002b.
—no goal
*four or more visits
**among those whose delivery was non-institutional
NA=not applicable

Care during pregnancy

No more than two in three pregnant women availed of an antenatal check-up, only 44 per cent reported three or more antenatal check-up visits, and only one-third underwent a check-up within the first trimester of pregnancy (IIPS and ORC Macro, 2000). Some two-third (66.8 per cent) of recently delivered women had obtained two or more tetanus-toxoid injections and just less than one half (47.5 per cent) had received a three-month supply of iron and folic acid supplements. In fact, only 20 per cent received all the recommended antenatal care services.

Wide state-wise variation is evident (IIPS and ORC Macro, 2000). In such states as Bihar, Nagaland, Rajasthan and Uttar Pradesh, for example, fewer than 10 per cent received all the recommended services. The southern states, in contrast, fared better, and in such states as Goa, Kerala and Tamil Nadu, more than half had received all recommended services. Likewise, variation is observed in the proportions receiving care within the first trimester, ranging from 15 per cent in Bihar to 81 per cent in Kerala.

Antenatal care tends to be perceived as unnecessary and to be availed only in case of health complications. Nationally, for example, of the 35 per cent of recently delivered women who received no antenatal care, the main reason cited by almost two-thirds was that this was unnecessary or not customary. In comparison, some 15 per cent cited cost and 9 per cent cited lack of permission from the family (IIPS and ORC Macro, 2000). A more in-depth case study of pregnancy-related experiences in three states (Andhra Pradesh, Madhya Pradesh and Orissa) reports that 18 per cent of women who suffered complications in pregnancy (and survived) did not seek care: the main reasons cited were that the problem was not serious (27 per cent) or that "the problem would go away" (16 per cent) (Murthy and Barua, 2001). Other studies suggest that women who experienced a morbidity during pregnancy and sought care were considerably more likely to opt for care from the private sector, including unqualified practitioners, rather than access free government services (Bhatia, 1995; Griffiths and Stephenson, 2001).

Smaller studies suggest that among women who received antenatal care, visits tended to be motivated by a perceived health complication rather than as a routine requirement of pregnancy. For example, a study in the slums of Delhi reveals that while 91 per cent of women availed of antenatal care, and an average of three visits were made, a large proportion of these visits were motivated by a health complication; routine monitoring accounted for no more than one-third of all first and second visits and the first contact was typically made in the fifth or sixth month of pregnancy

(Bhandari and Mayank, 1999). There are, however, exceptions: studies in rural Karnataka, Tamil Nadu and Pondicherry suggest that large proportions of women did indeed receive timely antenatal care within the first trimester and were not motivated by perceived health problems (Matthews et al., 2001; Srinivasa et al., 1997).

Whatever the motive for seeking care, there is evidence that women who received no antenatal care were considerably more likely to die of maternal causes than women who had three or more antenatal contacts (Ganatra, Coyaji and Rao, 1998, case control study in Maharashtra). The stillbirth and perinatal mortality rate were reportedly lower and birth weight higher among women who received antenatal care compared to those who did not (Aras, Pai and Purandare, 1990; Kapoor, Reddaiah and Lobo, 1985). Moreover, women who made regular antenatal visits were more likely to initiate breastfeeding promptly and feed colostrum to their infants than other women (Nielsen et al., 1998).

Skilled attendance at delivery

As obstetric emergencies are largely unpredictable and can occur during labour, childbirth and the immediate postpartum period, emphasis on early detection of complications, skilled attendance at delivery and referral and treatment in cases of obstetric emergencies are the core of essential obstetric care. Skilled attendance at delivery has been identified as the single most effective measure required to reduce maternal mortality. Corroborating this link, one case-control study in rural Maharashtra reports that women who delivered in institutions or who were delivered by a trained attendant were twice as likely to survive than those who delivered at home or were delivered by untrained attendants (odds ratios of 2.02 and 1.9 respectively, Ganatra, Coyaji and Rao, 1996).

What is clear is that despite ongoing efforts of the family welfare programme, skilled attendance at delivery eludes most women. The situation has improved only modestly over the course of the 1990s—in 1998-99, fewer than half of all recent deliveries

(42 per cent) were assisted by a health professional, including 30 per cent by a doctor or nurse, and 11 per cent by an auxiliary nurse-midwife, a nurse, midwife or lady health visitor compared with 34 per cent of births delivered by trained attendants six years earlier. Over the same period, institutional deliveries increased from one in four births (25.5 per cent) to one in three (34 per cent), (IIPS, 1995; IIPS and ORC Macro, 2000).

While the proportion of births that take place institutionally may have increased, this increase is attributed to the private rather than the public sector. For example, in 1992-93, some 11 per cent of all recent births took place in private maternity facilities (hospitals and "nursing homes"); this percentage increased to 17 per cent by 1998-99. Over the same period, institutional births at public facilities remained almost constant—15 per cent and 16 per cent in 1992-93 and 1998-99, respectively (IIPS, 1995; IIPS and ORC Macro, 2000). Hence, although there has been an 8 per cent rise in institutional births, the increase in the private sector has been three times greater than in the public sector. This trend marks the failure of the public sector in providing essential health care, but also implies that the poor, who can ill afford private maternity care, are less likely than others to avail of institutional delivery facilities.

State-wise variation is wide. In Assam, Bihar, Meghalaya and Uttar Pradesh, fewer than one quarter of all recent deliveries were assisted by a skilled attendant compared to over 80 per cent so delivered in Tamil Nadu (84 per cent), Goa (91 per cent) and Kerala (94 per cent). Only some eight states reported that 50 per cent or more births were institutionally delivered. Smaller studies suggest that skilled attendance levels are even lower in some settings: for example a study in two districts of Uttar Pradesh (Sitapur and Agra) reports that 75 per cent or more births were delivered at home and assisted by untrained providers; available clinics and staff lacked proper equipment, supplies and knowledge to handle obstetric complications (Anonymous, 2001).

Studies suggest a close correspondence between antenatal care and skilled attendance at delivery. Multivariate analysis of NFHS data from rural Andhra Pradesh, Bihar, Gujarat and Rajasthan suggests that after controlling for other factors, women who received antenatal care were 2 to 5 times more likely to give birth in a medical institution than those who received no antenatal care (Sugathan, Mishra and Retherford, 2001). A smaller study of low to middle income women in urban Uttar Pradesh corroborates this link: women who had sought antenatal care were four times more likely than those who did not to seek trained attendance at delivery (Bloom, Lippeveld and Wypij, 1999). These findings suggest that it is possible to encourage skilled attendance at birth through the promotion of antenatal check-ups and related counselling.

Postpartum care

In India, where cultural conditions in some settings prohibit both the mother and child from leaving the house in the first 40 days after delivery, it is unlikely that postpartum care will be sought without the active engagement of the health sector by way of home visits and/or efforts at community mobilisation. Indeed, until recently, programmes intended to make pregnancy safer paid scant attention to the postpartum period. It is only recently that the Reproductive and Child Health Programme recommended three postpartum visits. However, it is notable that while the Tenth Plan goals cover antenatal and intra-partum care, not a single goal refers to the need to ensure adequate postpartum care.

In reality, postpartum care is rarely sought and if sought, is rarely comprehensive. Nationally, among women who underwent a non-institutional delivery in the three years prior to investigation, only 17 per cent obtained a postpartum check-up within two months, and only 2 per cent obtained a check-up within two days of birth. Of these, just one-third reported an abdominal examination (35 per cent), and around two-fifths reported receiving breast-feeding advice and baby care advice (43 per cent and 46 per cent respectively); even fewer (27 per cent) were counselled about family planning (IIPS and ORC Macro, 2000). In Bihar, Gujarat, Rajasthan and Uttar Pradesh, 10 per cent or fewer women whose births were non-institutional received any postpartum care up to two months following delivery. A more in-depth study of pregnancy-related experiences in three states (Andhra Pradesh, Madhya Pradesh and Orissa) confirms that postpartum contacts with providers were far from the norm irrespective of whether the woman died of maternal causes or survived with and without complications: indeed, the fact that a somewhat larger percentage of those who died of maternal causes obtained postpartum care than others (42 per cent versus 30 per cent) only suggests that care is sought in case of an emergency and not as a rule (Murthy and Barua, 2001).

Findings from NFHS clearly suggest that women whose non-institutional deliveries were attended by a doctor, nurse, midwife or lady health visitor were substantially more likely to obtain timely postpartum care (42 per cent) than those delivered by a dai (traditional birth attendant) or other untrained attendants (11 and 14 per cent respectively) (IIPS and ORC Macro, 2000). Moreover, women who survived pregnancy were considerably more likely to have had at least three antenatal check-ups and been visited by an auxiliary nurse-midwife during pregnancy (Murthy and Barua, 2001).

Of serious concern, in this scenario, is evidence from a variety of settings suggesting that women who experienced postpartum morbidity were unlikely to seek care on their own unless the morbidity was perceived to be life threatening; cost, lack of awareness of the consequences and the perception that morbidities are self-limiting were leading reasons (Bhandari and Mayank, 1999; Murthy and Barua, 2001; Srinivasa et al., 1997).

Unsafe abortion practices

It is estimated that roughly five to six million abortions continue to be performed annually; of these, only about 0.6 million abortions are performed in registered facilities while another estimated four to five million occur outside (Ganatra, 2000). Government facilities are clearly inadequate, and even when women are aware of the availability of services, the fact that services are skewed towards urban areas places a huge barrier to access among rural women. Young and unmarried women fare worst, and frequently resort to second trimester abortions from unqualified providers.

Recent amendments in the Medical Termination of Pregnancy Act are intended to facilitate mechanisms for the registration of centres and thereby increase the availability of registered facilities. Thus far, however, as reported above, complications resulting from unsafe abortion constitute a major source of reproductive mortality and morbidity: an estimated 12,000 abortion-related deaths occur annually, constituting 8 per cent of all maternal deaths (RGI, 2000). Also disturbing is the trend towards second trimester abortions, indicative of the widespread practice of sex-selective abortions and its likely contribution to morbidity.

Care of the newborn

Complications of childbirth continue to have a significant impact on the newborn, and almost 30 per cent of neonatal deaths are observed to have occurred as a result of injuries sustained during delivery (Kusiako, Ronsmans and van der Paal, 2000). Essential care of the newborn has been a part of maternal and child health services since the Child Survival and Safe Motherhood Programme introduced resuscitation, prevention of hypothermia and infection, promotion of breastfeeding and referral of sick newborns as part of the programme in 1992 (Singh and Paul, 1997). The Reproductive and Child Health Programme further enlarged and decentralised the newborn health component. First referral units were equipped, for example, to handle sick newborns as well as to provide emergency obstetric services. Training of paediatricians and nurses in neonatal resuscitation, begun in 1990, provides a uniform approach to neonatal resuscitation. While subsequent declines in neonatal mortality have been moderate, there is evidence that asphyxia-related deaths have declined significantly (Deorari et al., 2000).

Like postpartum care, neonatal health seeking is constrained by traditional practices that forbid newly delivered women from leaving the home and the health system's failure to provide home-based care in this period (Rama Rao et al., 2001). One study shows for example, that in a rural setting of Maharashtra, while 54 per cent of neonates studied had symptoms requiring care, only 3 per cent had actually sought care (Bang et al., 2001). Indeed, in view of the fact that many rural women continue to lack skilled attendance at delivery, home-based care of neonates is as important in the short term as enhancing access to first referral units. A study of home care in 39 villages in Maharashtra shows, for example, a 50 per cent reduction in neonatal mortality when home-based care was provided by trained providers, demonstrating that village health workers can be trained to handle complications at home (Bang et al., 1999). Clearly teaching village health personnel to detect, treat or refer on time is essential and has proved to be an effective way of addressing neonatal complications.

Individual and community level obstacles underlying pregnancy-related care

Utilisation of pregnancy-related health care services is undoubtedly influenced by such contextual factors as poverty and education (see, for example, IIPS and ORC Macro, 2000). What is clear is that women experiencing symptoms of morbidity do not always avail of services, and many women who seek care do not do so promptly, encounter difficulties in physically accessing services or face serious breakdowns in service at the facility level. Resulting delays in seeking appropriate care have been noted as the three critical delays that inhibit safe motherhood (Thaddeus and Maine, 1994). Several obstacles to prompt health care utilisation have been identified.

Lack of awareness of good pregnancy-related practices

Pregnant women, their families, and indeed the communities in which they live by and large have not yet recognised the need for skilled attendance at delivery or the array of skills that a birth attendant needs. For example, despite the relative proximity to health care facilities, women in rural Karnataka preferred to deliver at home (Ganapathy, Ramakrishna and Matthews, 2000). Pregnant women in Delhi similarly preferred to deliver at home and without trained attendants despite the availability of government, private and NGO-run hospitals (Mayank et al., 2001). In both studies, calling a nurse or doctor, or going to a hospital were deemed necessary only in case of complications.

Misperceptions abound. For example, as mentioned earlier, the use of pregnancy-related services is considered unnecessary (IIPS, 1995). Likewise, beliefs and practices regarding food during pregnancy, both on how much and what to eat, tend to encourage "eating down"—reducing women's already meagre average daily food intake and discouraging the intake of such nutritional items as meat and leafy vegetables—during pregnancy (Hutton, 1996; Nag, 1994; Ramachandran, 1989). Postpartum haemorrhage in many parts of western India is perceived to signify cleansing the body of bad blood and hence no cause for alarm (Ganatra and Hirve, 1995).

Danger signals are poorly understood. For example, a study in rural Karnataka concludes that poor understanding of the urgency of many intra-partum complications inhibited timely care seeking (Ganapathy, Ramakrishna and Matthews, 2000). A study of women in the slums of Delhi reports that among women who experienced bleeding during pregnancy, 44 per cent actually recognised it as a danger signal; of those experiencing high blood pressure, and swelling of the hands, face and feet, only 33 per cent and 9 per cent respectively, recognised its severity. Indeed, this study concludes that although the vast majority of pregnant women received antenatal care, fewer than 10 per cent had been informed about danger signals. Correspondingly, care seeking among those experiencing morbidity was far from universal—of those experiencing vaginal bleeding and high blood pressure during pregnancy, as many as 29 per cent and 21 per cent did not seek care; and for such conditions as anaemia, urinary symptoms, swelling and abnormal vaginal discharge, fewer than one-third actually sought care (Mayank et al., 2001). A comparison of the experiences of women who died in pregnancy (through verbal autopsies) with those who experienced and did not experience complications in three states (Andhra Pradesh, Madhya Pradesh and Orissa) suggests that awareness was largely experience based, and that those who suffered no complications were considerably less likely to be aware of danger signals than others (Murthy and Barua, 2001).

Despite misperceptions and lack of awareness of danger signals, provider-client interactions fail to build awareness, as reported, for example, by women who gave birth in the three years preceding investigation (IIPS and ORC Macro, 2000). Appropriate diet was discussed with just over half of these women; while the danger signals of pregnancy, information on delivery, newborn care and family planning were explained to between one quarter and two-fifths (36, 41, 38, 28 per cent respectively). Small studies suggest an even more disturbing situation. For example, a study of women in the slums of Delhi reports that only 43 per cent were provided information on appropriate diet; far fewer were given information on breastfeeding (5 per cent), subsequent contraception (4 per cent), and the importance of delivering in hospitals and of postnatal check-ups (28 per cent and 4 per cent, respectively). Only 4 per cent were informed of danger signals (Bhandari and Mayank, 1999). A prospective study of pregnant women in rural Karnataka similarly reports that only 44 per cent were informed about appropriate diet in pregnancy; and even fewer were advised about breastfeeding, danger signals or the need for postpartum check-ups (10 per cent) or informed about contraception (12 per cent) (Matthews et al., 2001). Compliance with antenatal treatment, such as consumption of iron and folic acid supplements, may be considerably influenced by the kind of counselling that women receive on their advantages and disadvantages; a small study cites the failure of health workers to provide regular and detailed counselling on the benefits and mechanisms of these supplements as a key factor underlying women's lack of compliance (Tuladhar et al., 1997).

As a result of continued misperceptions, where care is sought, it occurs, in all likelihood, as a last resort, among women whose symptoms are particularly severe and unresponsive to home remedies. Lack of information on the location of appropriate facilities can, in these circumstances, exacerbate fatal outcomes: for example, compared to women who survived an obstetric complication, many who died sought emergency care from facilities that were not adequately equipped to provide such care (Ganatra, Coyaji and Rao, 1998).

Women's lack of decision-making authority

Where women's decision-making is restricted and women's illness lies low on the family priority list, decisions regarding health care for pregnancy and pregnancy-related complications are frequently delayed, often with dire health consequences (Gittelsohn et al., 1994; Jeffery, Jeffery and Lyons, 1989). Even educated women are not always likely to be the main decision-maker when sick (Ganatra and Hirve, 1995; Ganatra, Coyaji, and Rao, 1998). In the slums of Delhi, for example, as many as 81 per cent of pregnant women required permission from other family members such as her husband and mother-in-law to avail of antenatal or delivery care, even in the case of an emergency (Bhandari and Mayank, 1999). An in-depth case study of pregnancy-related experiences in Andhra Pradesh, Madhya Pradesh and Orissa reports that 9 per cent of women experiencing complications in the postpartum stage were denied care by family members; and of those who sought care, only 13 per cent of those experiencing complications and 26 per cent of those who did not experience complications made the decision to seek care themselves (Murthy and Barua, 2001).

Women's restricted mobility compounds this delay in seeking appropriate care. In many parts of India, strict seclusion norms inhibit contact with the health sector. For example, one study of women in Uttar Pradesh and Tamil Nadu observes that only about 38 per cent and 44 per cent of women from each state can visit a health centre unescorted (Jejeebhoy, 2000b). Another study of women who had given birth in the three years preceding the investigation in Varanasi shows that after controlling for such factors as age, education and household structure, women with greater mobility were more likely than others to obtain antenatal and delivery care, and suggests that mobility is as important as such better known determinants as education in influencing appropriate pregnancy-related care seeking (Bloom, Wypij and Das Gupta, 2001). Financial and opportunity costs further limit women's access to health care. In general, families, including women themselves, spend less time, effort and money seeking health care for women and girls than for men (Chatterjee, 1996) and women are unlikely to have independent control over the resources required to seek care (see for example, Jejeebhoy, 2000b). Women's illness ranks low among family priorities, especially when the condition is perceived as non-threatening or self-limiting, thus delaying the decision to seek care (Ganatra and Hirve, 1995; Thaddeus and Maine, 1994): Similarly, in Andhra Pradesh, Madhya Pradesh and Orissa, women who did not seek care for complications experienced during pregnancy cited lack of mobility and lack of resources as reasons while those who did not seek care for complications experienced in the postpartum stage cited lack of resources as the reason (Murthy and Barua, 2001).

The finding of a case-control study in Maharashtra that women who delivered in their parental homes were significantly less likely to die than women who delivered in their husband's home (odds ratios 0.4) highlights the enormity of women's powerlessness in their marital homes. Evidently parents are far more likely to make timely health interventions in, and are far readier to incur expenses on saving the lives of their daughters and sisters than on their daughters-in-law and wives (Ganatra, Coyaji and Rao, 1998).

Son preference and the resulting disparities in health care and feeding practices of children have been well documented in India. Most studies suggest that gender disparities in infant mortality become apparent from the post-neonatal stage, and indeed the NFHS confirms this (IIPS and ORC Macro, 2000). However, small and in-depth studies do suggest that gender disparities operate even at the neonatal level. A study in Salem district, rural Tamil Nadu, suggests that female neonatal deaths were significantly higher among multiparous women with no surviving sons than primiparous women (Nielsen et al., 1997).

Role of men in maternity care

Men have traditionally remained uninformed about their wives' pregnancy-related experiences and needs, yet are significant decision-makers with regard to pregnancy-related care and expenditure. For example, in one study in north India, men justify the central role they play in health care choices for women. "It is the husband or elder male members of the family who decide where or to which clinic women should be taken. Women have no freedom in such matters but men have all the freedom and power to decide" (Khan, Khan and Mukerjee, 1997). However, their decisions can be uninformed as few are aware of the danger signals their wives might experience.

Evidence suggests however that men are interested and do want to be more involved, and that programmes have largely neglected to involve them in pregnancy-related matters. For example, a qualitative case study of young couples in Gujarat and West Bengal reports that while most men accompanied their wives to health facilities during pregnancy, some expressed their hesitation. Men also reported that they provided physical and emotional support to their wives during pregnancy and the postpartum period but reported that in conformity with prevailing gender norms, "I do it secretly. Because it is shameful" (Santhya et al., 2003). A recent study conducted in Delhi reveals that more than 80 per cent of pregnant women and their husbands wanted husbands to participate in maternity care; moreover, when permitted, 60 per cent of their husbands attended antenatal clinics with their wives. This study confirms, moreover, that couple counselling in the antenatal and postpartum periods was positively associated with postpartum family planning acceptance (Varkey et al., 2001).

Domestic violence

Significant proportions of pregnant women experience domestic violence. A facility-based study of some 800 women reported that 21 per cent had experienced abuse during pregnancy, and compared to other women, were more likely to report unplanned pregnancy, receive inadequate antenatal care and be poorly educated (Muthal-Rathore, Tripathi and Arora, 2002). There are indications that women who experience domestic violence are also more likely than other women to report foetal and infant deaths, attributed in part to their compromised care seeking (Jejeebhoy, 1998a). Indeed, there is a suggestion that death due to domestic violence may be a pregnancy-related cause of death that is frequently overlooked in discussions of maternal health. A study in rural Maharashtra observes that deaths from such causes as drowning, poisoning, hanging and burns could be a result of domestic violence. If these cases had been included in the definition of maternal deaths, they would have accounted for some 16 per cent of maternal deaths obtained in a community-based survey, and 13 per cent of those obtained in a hospital-based survey (Ganatra, Coyaji and Rao, 1998).

Failure to provide comprehensive pregnancy-related services

As mentioned earlier, recommended antenatal services include three or more antenatal visits to monitor the progress of the pregnancy and detect complications; however, few women report obtaining the entire array of services. The recent NFHS 2, for example, shows that among women who gave birth in the three years preceding the survey, in only about half of all visits were weight and blood pressure checked, blood tested and abdomen palpated (IIPS and ORC Macro, 2000). Smaller studies reveal similar findings. In the slums of Delhi for example, blood pressure was recorded among 75 per cent of women who made antenatal visits, abdominal and vaginal examinations were conducted among 56 per cent and 20 per cent, respectively; blood and urine tested among 60 per cent, and weight and height recorded among 61 per cent and 8 per cent respectively (Bhandari and Mayank, 1999). In rural Karnataka, while almost all the women (>95 per cent) reported receiving tetanus-toxoid injections and iron and folic acid supplements, 81 per cent had their abdomen palpated, and 40-60 per cent reported blood pressure reading, blood and urine analysis and weight monitoring (Matthews et al., 2001).

Poor quality of care

Pregnancy related care is provided largely in the public sector in India. Although poor quality of care is rarely cited by women as a reason for not availing antenatal services in the public sector, the shift towards increased private sector deliveries suggests that perceived quality of care may indeed play a role in inhibiting access to pregnancy-related care from the public sector. At the same time, regulatory systems for pricing and monitoring quality of services in the private sector remain unclear.

Poor quality of care also appears to inhibit institutional deliveries or deliveries by public health personnel. Health workers are often unavailable or unwilling to attend deliveries in home settings (Ganapathy, Ramakrishna and Matthews, 2000). Providers may be unsympathetic, and display attitudes that label women as dirty or ignorant (Jeffery, Jeffery and Lyon, 1989; Ram, 1994). Staff at facilities do not give women sufficient information or time, or explain the course of medication prescribed (Bhandari and Mayank, 1999). A few studies report women's preference for traditional birth attendants as they are perceived to be more supportive (Ganapathy, Ramakrishna and Matthews, 2000; Jeffery, Jeffery and Lyon, 1989).

Lack of accessible appropriate facilities

Distance and the unavailability of public transportation are common constraints to health care utilisation, especially in rural areas, and play an important role in inhibiting timely access to institutional delivery (Thaddeus and Maine, 1994). A case control study in Maharashtra observes that delay in seeking care, measured as the time lag between onset of symptoms and reaching the first health contact, was one of the most significant factors increasing the risk of dying (Ganatra, Coyaji and Rao, 1998). The study observes that pregnant women who died from obstetric complications travelled further and took longer to reach first or final contact facilities than women who survived such complications. In this study, 26 per cent of all deaths occurred within the home, 18 per cent occurred en route to a facility, and 20 per cent occurred in facilities that were not equipped to attend to obstetric complications. Only one in three women who died (36 per cent) were able to reach an appropriately equipped facility. Women with access to timely care—as measured by the number of facilities visited before an appropriate facility was reached, the presence of an auxiliary nurse-midwife in the village and trained attendance at delivery—were significantly less likely to die than other women (Ganatra, Coyaji and Rao, 1998). A study in rural Haryana corroborates the link between accessibility and mortality; it notes that villages with a health care centre reported significantly lower levels of perinatal mortality and significantly higher levels of health service utilisation than those with only a subcentre or no facilities (Kumar, Singh and Kaur, 1997). An in-depth case study of pregnancy-related experiences in Andhra Pradesh, Madhya Pradesh and Orissa reports that lack of accessible facilities inhibited 18 per cent of pregnant women from seeking care for complications experienced at delivery and 15 per cent from seeking care in the postpartum stage; lack of transport was cited by 9 per cent in each group (Murthy and Barua, 2001).

Affordability of services

Affordability can also inhibit timely access to care although few studies have addressed this link in India. While services may be theoretically free of cost, frequently medicine, blood and even transportation costs can delay access to a medical facility. For example, the fact that surviving a complication is costly is demonstrated in a case control study in Andhra Pradesh: findings reveal that the average amount spent by families of women who survived a complication was nearly twice as high as that incurred by families of women who died (Murthy and Barua, 2001).

Programme related obstacles

Programme actions to make pregnancy safer

Maternal and newborn health has been on the national agenda for several decades but has undergone significant shifts in programme emphasis. Between the 1960s and the early 1990s, programmes stressed antenatal care and the high-risk approach. During this period, notably in the Fifth Five-year Plan (1974-79), maternal and child health and nutrition programmes were integrated with family planning services. The failure of the risk approach to support women who develop complications of delivery is well-known, and in keeping with the worldwide recognition of the importance of emergency obstetric care and the necessary referral network that such care implies, in the early 1990s, programmes aimed at pregnancy-related care shifted focus to the provision of essential and emergency obstetric care, notably, early registration of pregnancy, provision of at least three antenatal check-ups, provision of skilled attendance at delivery preferably in the context of institutional births and provision of three postpartum visits. In addition, special measures for neonatal care included detection, referral and management of high-risk cases such as low birth and premature babies and treatment of asphyxia.

The Child Survival and Safe Motherhood Programme, launched in 1992, was the first to mark this shift in emphasis. It combined maternal with child health interventions. Key strategies of the Child Survival and Safe Motherhood Programme relating to pregnancy-related and neonatal care include (a) the establishment of first referral units within existing community health centres to provide emergency obstetric care; (b) efforts to improve maternal care at the village level including immunisation, and the identification and referral of high-risk cases; (c) increased access to village level care through better trained auxiliary nurse-midwives and continued training of traditional birth attendants; (d) upgrading equipment and providing drugs at the subcentre level; and (e) introducing measures to raise awareness of safe pregnancy-related practices at the community level (Mavalankar, 1999b). However, the programme had several limitations. Training tended to focus on child survival and neglected maternal health, including the importance of emergency obstetric care; and first referral units remained poorly equipped and staffed—not even half of these units were fully functional by the late 1990s and few had regular access to supplies of blood. Identification of high-risk mothers and complications during pregnancy tended to be uneven and community awareness building was limited (Mavalankar, 1999b).

The Reproductive and Child Health Programme, launched in 1997, built on this experience and made a special effort to strengthen emergency obstetric facilities and care of the newborn at the district level. The National Population Policy 2000 (MOHFW, 2000) and the Tenth Five-year Plan (Planning Commission, 2002b) further underscored measures to reduce maternal and newborn mortality, basically reinforcing the thrust of the Reproductive and Child Health Programme. Presently (late 2003) components of the second wave of the Reproductive and Child Health Programme are being finalised, incorporating new measures to achieve emergency obstetric and newborn care (MOHFW, 2003d).

Each programme and policy statement has set ambitious goals in terms of reducing maternal and infant mortality. However, these somewhat unrealistic goals have had to be continuously revised. For example, the Child Survival and Safe Motherhood Programme proposed achieving a maternal mortality ratio of 200 per 100,000 live births by the year 2000. This goal was revised by the Reproductive and Child Health Programme, which set itself the equally difficult goal of attaining a maternal mortality ratio below 100 per 100,000 live births by 2010, along with an infant mortality rate of 30 per 1,000 live births, and skilled attendance at all births (MOHFW, 2000; 2002b). The Tenth Plan (Planning Commission, 2002b) has further revised these goals and now aims to attain a maternal mortality ratio of 200 per 100,000 live births by the year 2007, along with a neonatal mortality rate of 26 per 1,000 live births and skilled attendance at 80 per cent of all births.

The Reproductive and Child Health Programme focuses its strategies to enhance maternal and newborn health in four broad areas, namely strengthening facilities and upgrading the skills of a variety of providers, enhancing institutional delivery and mobilising community support, promoting skilled attendance at home and the subcentre level, and advocating postpartum and essential newborn care (see MOHFW, 2003d).

Strengthening facilities and upgrading provider skills

The Reproductive and Child Health Programme seeks to strengthen essential and emergency obstetric care facilities at the sub-district and district level by expanding existing rural health services to include facilities for institutional delivery. The intention is to strengthen the network of primary health centres and subcentres as well as other government health facilities in rural areas, and government or municipal hospitals and health posts in urban areas. A total of 1,748 first referral units, usually housed in community health centres, are to be strengthened and are to provide comprehensive essential and emergency obstetric and newborn care, including 24-hour normal delivery services, assisted vaginal deliveries, as well as blood storage facilities. Related reproductive health services, such as family planning counselling, supply of contraceptives, conduct of abortions and STI/RTI diagnosis and treatment are also to be provided. In addition, arrangements have been made in both rural and urban areas for expanding access, as part of the public health system, to the services of a sizeable private sector (maternity homes, hospitals and physicians) and, in some areas, NGOs. Attention is also to be paid to ensuring that supplies of medicines are regular and that appropriate equipment is available and functioning.

Measures have been taken, moreover, to fill the dearth of trained providers at the facility and community levels. At first referral units in which specialists are not available, the services of private gynaecologists and anaesthesiologists will be contracted to provide services on a regular basis. Likewise, provision is made for the deployment of additional nurses where necessary. Training needs have also been recognised. State governments are expected to enhance provider skills through on-the-job training and create a pool of trained community level skilled birth attendants (IIPS and ORC Macro, 2000; MOHFW, 2000).

The Tenth Plan (2002-07) endorses these strategies. It underscores the need to enhance the number of functioning first referral units/community health centres by (a) posting specialists (obstetricians, gynaecologists and paediatricians) in these facilities; (b) providing funds for hiring specialists, including anaesthesiologists on a contract basis; (c) improving access to blood banks; and (d) establishing links with private and NGO sector institutions in providing essential and emergency obstetric care. Round-the-clock delivery services are to be available in 50 per cent of all primary health centres in addition to all community health centres, first referral units and district hospitals; and emergency obstetric care is to be available at all first referral units and district hospitals. Finally, it advocates that at least one trained traditional birth attendant must be available in each village, and must receive training in clean delivery practices (MOHFW, 2002b; Planning Commission, 2002b).

The draft Reproductive and Child Health Programme-2 (to be implemented in 2004) similarly advocates enhancing provider skills and expanding the pool of physicians. It goes beyond earlier programmes by advocating that general physicians be trained in anaesthesiology and caesarean delivery skills, and general surgeons be involved in caesarean-section deliveries at first referral units and district hospitals. It also recommends establishing blood storage facilities at all first referral units and blood banks at all district hospitals.

Enhancing institutional delivery and mobilising community support

The Reproductive and Child Health Programme incorporates measures intended to mobilise women and communities to seek institutional deliveries. These include attempts to ensure early registration of pregnancy (by 16 weeks); provide advice on appropriate diet, rest and danger signals during pregnancy and encourage institutional deliveries. The programme seeks, moreover, to engage community support for the timely transport of women with complications to first referral units.

The Tenth Plan and the Reproductive and Child Health Programme-2 propose to strengthen this component. The Tenth Plan seeks to ensure the availability of transport for pregnant women to reach referral facilities by involving the community and ensuring dedicated funds. The Reproductive and Child Health Programme-2 proposes moreover that monetary incentives be provided to traditional birth attendants, anganwadi workers and other village-level workers to accompany pregnant women to institutions for delivery; make funds available for the transportation of expectant mothers for routine deliveries and emergency obstetric care; and cover the expenses incurred by poor women (below the poverty line) on delivery and emergency obstetric services at recognised private facilities. At the same time, social mobilisation efforts are advocated that will enhance the demand for institutional deliveries and referral of women with complications. Educating communities on danger signals and good practices is also proposed.

Promoting skilled attendance at birth at home and subcentre levels

The Reproductive and Child Health Programme recognises the need, at the same time, to promote skilled attendance at delivery at home or in subcentres. The programme advocates several measures to enable contact between pregnant women and providers from an early stage of pregnancy and referral for hospital delivery in cases of complications. These include ensuring at least three antenatal visits (at a clinic or through outreach) and providing services to manage and refer high-risk cases, detect and treat anaemia, monitor blood pressure, distribute iron and folic acid supplements and administer two doses of tetanus-toxoid injections, awareness raising on risk factors, breastfeeding, and rest and nutrition. Auxiliary-nurse midwives and traditional birth attendants who have been trained in clean delivery practices are expected to attend births taking place in the home, as well as identify high-risk cases and ensure their timely referral.

The draft Reproductive and Child Health Programme-2 further strengthens this component. As before, it reiterates the need, where institutional delivery is not possible, for the promotion of deliveries by auxiliary nurse-midwives/nurses at subcentres or homes. It proposes, in addition, to train a group of women as 'community skilled birth attendants', who will be drawn from among the better educated women residents of each village, who, once trained, will be given assistance in setting up facilities to provide pregnancy-related care and referral. It needs to be noted that while the training needs of medical officers and auxiliary nurse-midwives have not been fully met, plans are underway to train a whole new cadre of providers whose services may be inaccessible to the poor since they are fee-based. The feasibility of such a strategy needs to be carefully examined.

Postpartum and essential newborn care

A weak area in family welfare programmes has been the failure to address postpartum care. The Reproductive and Child Health Programme makes a significant attempt to address this gap. It advocates at least three postpartum visits, iron supplements for lactating mothers and the detection and treatment of anaemia, outreach care within 24 hrs of delivery by an auxiliary nurse-midwife, and treatment of puerperal sepsis. It also advocates essential newborn care including the operationalisation of district newborn care and home-based neonatal care, and the promotion of timely and exclusive breastfeeding. Other recommended services include the detection and referral of high-risk neonates, immunisation, treatment of asphyxia and the management of low birth weight babies at the community level. The Reproductive and Child Health Programme-2 refines this thrust by recommending the timing of postpartum visits—on days 1 and 7 and then at 6 weeks, with appropriate links for neonates.

Programme-level obstacles underlying pregnancy-related care

Thus far, there has not been a comprehensive mid-term or final assessment of the implementation and effectiveness of ongoing programmes. Preliminary assessments however are not encouraging (see for example, Mavalankar, 2003). Some points of issue are discussed in this section.

Skewed programme emphasis

The emphasis of maternal and child health programmes is skewed at many levels. Over the past few decades, maternal and child health services have been neglected due to programme emphasis on meeting family planning targets and the thrust towards universal immunisation (1980s) and polio eradication (1990s). Consequently, auxiliary nurse-midwives and medical officers have been more committed to meeting targets than providing pregnancy-related care. The lack of emphasis on recording maternal deaths has resulted in a lack of accountability. Strategies advocated in the Reproductive and Child Health Programme have not been uniformly implemented. Only a few primary health centres and community health centres provide the entire range of recommended services, or have upgraded facilities and hired additional trained staff (see Mavalankar, 2003 for a review). Even within maternal and child health interventions, the provision of services has been skewed, focusing more on the administration of tetanus-toxoid injections and iron and folic acid supplements than other activities (ICMR, 1997).

Despite the fact that HIV has begun to be observed among pregnant women seeking antenatal care and has reached over 1 per cent in several states, and despite preliminary evidence from pilot programmes that voluntary counselling, testing and treatment may be acceptable to pregnant women (Bultreys et al., 2002), neither the issue of integrating HIV counselling nor the provision of anti-retroviral therapy to women attending antenatal clinics has received attention in the design of safe motherhood programmes.

Lack of trained staff at facilities

Staffing at facilities is limited. A facility survey conducted in 1999 reports that obstetricians/gynaecologists were available in only 78 per cent of district hospitals, 48 per cent of first referral units and 28 per cent of community health centres. Even nurses were not available in 6 per cent of district hospitals, 7 per cent of first referral units and 13 per cent of community health centres (IIPS, 2001b). A 1998 review of government rural health infrastructure suggests that at the national level, considerable shortfalls exist: against the norm of one auxiliary nurse-midwife per subcentre, 17 per cent of subcentres remain under-staffed; and against a norm of four specialists per community health centre, 68 per cent remain under-staffed (Jesani, 2001). As all staff members do not reside in the area where they are posted, health services are unlikely to be available round-the-clock as recommended (Mavalankar, 1999a). While the Reproductive and Child Health Programme advocates hiring of additional staff at remote or inaccessible subcentres and primary health centres and specialists on contract basis at under-staffed facilities, this has not proved successful as providers are presumably unwilling to serve in these settings (Mavalankar, 2003).

Unmet training needs

Training needs have clearly not been met and few medical officers and providers have been trained in public health. In 1999, only 19 per cent of medical officers at district hospitals, 17 per cent of those at first referral centres and 11 per cent of those at community health centres were trained in emergency obstetric care and a slightly larger proportion were trained in newborn care (21 per cent, 22 per cent and 17 per cent, respectively, IIPS, 2001b). Auxiliary nurse-midwives are so poorly trained that many are not adept at checking blood pressure or testing urine for sugar. Moreover, their training does not cover the practical skills needed for conducting delivery or the socio-behavioural aspects of health (Mavalankar, 1999a). The training needs of providers have not been addressed, particularly for the provision of emergency obstetric care, even under the Reproductive and Child Health Programme. Actual clinical maternity experience and skills for providing emergency obstetric care were assessed to be limited among a range of providers, including auxiliary nurse-midwives, lady health visitors, nurses and medical officers (Mother Care, 1996). A review of maternal and child health care use and the ability of the public sector to provide antenatal and emergency obstetric services reports that while blueprints for safe motherhood programmes exist, the technical competence of providers was limited and equipment unavailable, particularly with regard to emergency services (Rama Rao et al., 2001).

Poorly equipped facilities and non-availability of services

Few first referral units in practice provide the full range of services, particularly in high mortality settings due to lack of equipment, consumables and basic infrastructure, and poorly trained and complacent providers (GOI and European Commission, 2001; MOHFW, 2002b). For example, a survey of reproductive health care services in 23 districts of 14 states confirms that pregnant women who experienced complications during pregnancy were rarely provided appropriate emergency obstetric care at first referral units (ICMR, 1997).

Essential equipment and consumables are not routinely available in first referral units or even district hospitals (see for example, GOI and European Commission, 2001). For example, a facility survey conducted in 1999 reports that drug kits for emergency obstetric care were available in only 30 per cent of district hospitals, 29 per cent of first referral units and 15 per cent of community health centres. Even kits for normal delivery/labour room delivery were available in only 52 per cent, 68 per cent and 48 per cent of these facilities, respectively. Likewise, kits for newborn care were available in one-third and neonatal resuscitation equipment in about two-fifths of district hospitals and first referral units; only 15 per cent of community health centres had such equipment (IIPS, 2001b). The availability of banked blood is erratic; blood banks serve, on average, a population of 1.5-2 million at the district level. Inappropriate storage conditions and faulty equipment compound the problem (Mavalankar, 2003). There is also a concern that community-managed funds for emergency transport has been misused in some settings.

The way forward

Maternal mortality and morbidity vary considerably across the country but remain, in most states, unacceptably high and largely preventable. A variety of factors contribute to these high rates of morbidity, such as women's powerlessness in the decision-making process and a traditional reluctance to seek timely and skilled pregnancy-related care. Referral systems and facilities to deal with emergencies are rarely in place and quality of care tends to be insensitive to women's needs. Although the 1990s have witnessed increased programme commitment to enhancing reproductive health in general and pregnancy-related care in particular, implementation appears to have been erratic and training needs have not been met.

Wide schisms in pregnancy-related outcomes and care are evident across the country and are particularly adverse in the EAG states, which are in need of special programmatic attention.

The Reproductive and Child Health Programme document offers a blueprint for action, yet vast obstacles continue to impede its implementation. Indeed, it is unclear whether programmes will make a significant dent in maternal health services or in reducing maternal and neonatal mortality levels by 2007 as proposed.

The challenge now is to ensure that the second wave of the Reproductive and Child Health Programme is more responsive to women's needs. Further improvements in maternal outcomes will rest on efforts to improve the level of care among the most under-served—poor women with limited education, who live in poor neighbourhoods in rural areas, marry and initiate child-bearing early and have generally poor access to primary health care.

Programme recommendations

- Actions are required that apprise pregnant women and their families of danger signals and action required in case these are experienced, ways of negotiating appropriate care, nutrition and rest during pregnancy, and their right to avail of skilled and affordable attendance at birth. Efforts are needed that mobilise women, inform them of their rights, enable them to exert a voice in family affairs and make contingency plans for unforeseen pregnancy-related problems, and create among them a feeling of entitlement to health care and other services. These will involve short- and long-term strategies, multisectoral changes, and changes at the level of women, their families and service providers.

- Key of course is ensuring essential and emergency obstetric care and institutional deliveries. In the shorter term, ensuring trained attendance at delivery at home or the subcentre level is critical. Closer links need to be forged between the various levels of the health system, as well as between the formal and non-formal, public and private sector providers of care. Staff availability at the facility level and adequate training to staff are imperative. There is a need to explore whether mid-level providers and non-specialist medical officers can also be engaged, with due training, in the provision of maternal health services. Such options as enabling trained general physicians to provide emergency obstetric care including caesarean-sections deliveries and enabling trained auxiliary nurse-midwives to manage basic obstetric emergencies when doctors are not available (for example the provision of injectable antibiotics to treat postpartum infection or the provision of anti-hypertensive medication in cases of pre-eclampsia or uterine evacuations in cases of incomplete abortion) need serious consideration as a means of extending emergency obstetric care in rural areas (Mavalankar, 2002a). Effective partnerships with the private sector to ensure safe pregnancy outcomes may be yet another strategy for overcoming current shortages of trained staff.
- Given the large state-wide disparities in maternal and neonatal mortality and related care seeking, flexibility is required in designing programmes that are responsive to the contextual situation and needs of different states.
- Social mobilisation efforts to involve women, communities and elected leaders in making pregnancy safer have not been successful, and there is a suggestion that funds allotted for these activities may have been misused or under-used. Women's self-help groups could be strengthened to take on

the challenge of establishing mechanisms to ensure timely and appropriate care. However, the extent to which the provision of transport funds through panchayats/village level institutions and other innovations have been implemented and the constraints faced need to be better understood and acted upon.

- Quality of care needs should be addressed as women and families continue to be poorly informed about danger signals, birth planning and appropriate care, provider interaction tends to be unfriendly or threatening, and follow-up is limited, including in the critical postpartum period.
- Multi-pronged efforts are required to raise community awareness of the adverse health consequences of early marriage and pregnancy, and of legislation prohibiting marriage for girls under 18. Equally important are efforts that break the cycle of vulnerability and powerlessness in adolescence itself, such as, through the provision of livelihood skills and expanded life options to adolescent females. On the other hand, given the reality of persistent early marriage, it is important to ensure that adolescent girls who do experience pregnancy are physically fit to endure the demands of pregnancy and at the same time, train providers to provide services that recognise that pregnant adolescents are an extremely vulnerable group, both physically and socially.
- Where women's own decision-making and mobility are limited, the participation and awareness of husbands and other influential community members in ensuring safe motherhood are important, and need to be more actively sought. Misconceptions that health care during pregnancy is unnecessary must be confronted at the community level, and among pregnant women, their husbands and the families in which they reside. Pilot interventions have highlighted that men can be willing partners in pregnancy, and such interventions must be upscaled.

Research recommendations

Further improvements in maternal and neonatal outcomes are also hampered by limitations of evidence. Available research and evaluation studies conducted over the past decade have been largely small-scale and facility-based. Universal registration of births and deaths has not yet been achieved. Assessments of reproductive and child health programmes have not been undertaken. There remain huge gaps in what we know about maternal mortality and obstetric morbidity and programme implementation, constraints to good maternal and newborn health and the quality of services to meet their health needs. Moreover, the ways in which programme delivery models can overcome the powerful negative influence of gender inequity and women's, notably young women's, powerlessness, and at the same time facilitate the exercise of reproductive choice among women need urgent attention. We discuss below a few critical research needs.

- Evidence is needed on underlying risk factors that shed light on why pregnancy-related morbidity has been largely hospital-based. There is a paucity of community-based studies that examine the extent of maternal morbidity and its correlates. Evidence is needed on underlying risk factors, why women's obstetric health needs remain unmet, the array of constraints women face in seeking reproductive health care and the kinds of interventions that can be designed to respond to these needs at the family, community and service delivery levels.
- While women are generally under-served, among the most neglected group are adolescent girls. Research is required that focuses on their reproductive health needs, nutritional status, the risks of early marriage and childbearing, their powerlessness and how this attenuates their vulnerability in terms of timely health seeking during pregnancy and childbirth. Equally important is operations research that tests the feasibility of models intended to reduce the vulnerability of young women.

- Little research is available on the quality of pregnancy-related health care from the perspective of individual clients. Evidence is needed that assesses how women perceive the maternal health services available to them, their preference for the private sector and the kind of service adjustments that are necessary to attract more institutional deliveries in the public sector.
- Although access to maternal and newborn services is considerably influenced, in practice, by the cost of services, we know relatively little about expenditure patterns associated with pregnancy and childbirth and the extent to which cost factors inhibit timely health seeking and influence pregnancy-related outcomes. Although the private sector provides a considerable proportion of maternal and newborn health services, it remains difficult to assess how private sector maternity and newborn care is priced: records are poorly maintained and regulatory mechanisms do not stipulate public access to their accounts and there is little research on its functioning or the financial processes governing it. Direct and indirect estimates of the cost of maternal and newborn health services in the public and private sectors need to be established to improve cost efficiency and prevent misuse of costly processes.
- Unfortunately lessons from the Reproductive and Child Health Programme thus far are not available. Research or rigorous documentation is required that explores, in selected geographic settings, the extent to which measures have been implemented and the difficulties encountered, both in social mobilisation and in accessing skilled birth attendance. In effect, assessments of workable programme strategies and the kinds of modifications necessary, from the of perspectives women, the community and the health system are imperative in order that evidence-based adjustments in programmes can be effected.

Induced Abortion

K.G. Santhya and Shalini Verma

Despite the liberalisation of abortion services since the early 1970s, access to safe abortion services remains limited for the vast majority of Indian women, particularly in rural areas. An overwhelming proportion of induced abortions (6.7 million annually as per indirect estimate, see Chhabra and Nuna, 1994) take place in unauthorised centres, which provide services of varying degrees of safety. At the same time, in recent years significant changes in the abortion scenario have been taking place in the country, which have had wide ramifications.

The changing face of abortion

The period since the 1990s have witnessed major changes in the field of abortion including the adoption of new legislative measures, the introduction of new technologies and the growing demand for sex-selective abortion. Some of these developments, such as the recent amendments to the Medical Termination of Pregnancy Act and the introduction of innovative abortion technologies, such as the improved manual vacuum aspiration technique and medical abortion, are expected to increase the availability of safe abortion services. However, other trends, such as the growing demand for sex-selective abortion, are likely to increase the incidence of unsafe abortion and adversely change gender dynamics even further.

Legislative measures

Recognising the failure of the Medical Termination of Pregnancy (MTP) Act of 1972 to make legal abortions widely available, the government amended the Act in 2002. With the recent amendment, authority for the approval of registration of MTP centres has been decentralised from the state to the district level (Government of India, 2002; Mallik, 2002). Additionally, the Reproductive and Child Health Programme launched in 1997 and the National Population Policy, 2000 have delineated a number of strategies to increase access to safe abortion at the primary health care level (MOHFW, 2000).

Amendments have also been introduced in the Pre-natal Diagnostic Techniques (Regulation and Prevention of Misuse) (PNDT) Act of 1994. This was necessitated as the PNDT Act had failed to curb the practice of testing for sex determination and consequent sex-selective abortion in the country (Oomman and Ganatra, 2002). With the recent amendment to the PNDT Act, preconception and pre-implantation procedures for sex selection are banned in the country. The Amendment stipulates compulsory maintenance of written records by diagnostic centres/doctors offering sonography service. Local authorities have also been given powers to ensure the enforcement of the Act (Government of India, 2003; Mallik, 2002). With these measures, the government expects to prevent women from resorting to sex-selective abortions, which are conducted during the second-trimester and carry a high risk of complications for women.

Medical abortion

Medical abortion or abortion by orally administered regimens of mifepristone and misoprostol has recently been accepted worldwide as an effective and safe option for early abortion.

Clinical trials in a number of countries, including India, have shown that the use of the standard French regimen, which includes administering 600 mg of mifepristone during the first visit and 400 μg of misoprostol during a follow-up visit after two days, combined with a follow-up visit after two weeks, is effective in 95 per cent of the cases of early abortion (i.e., up to 49 days from the last menstrual period) and safe (major complications were reported in only 0.5 per cent of the cases) (Coyaji, 2002).

The Drug Controller of India has approved the use of medical abortion in April 2002 (Coyaji, 2002). Given the current situation in India, where abortion-related mortality and morbidity is high, medical abortion offers great potential for improving access to abortion and safety as it does not require extensive infrastructure and is non-invasive. Further, as the client does not need to be hospitalised, medical abortion offers women greater independence, control and privacy. However, the potential for misuse is a matter of concern. In fact, although abortion tablets are required to be sold by medical prescription and consumed under medical supervision, these pills are reportedly widely available over-the-counter and unsupervised consumption is rising (*Times of India*, 2002; *Hindustan Times*, 2003; *India Today*, 2003). Plans to develop national guidelines to introduce abortion pills in the family welfare programme are currently under discussion.

Apart from initial clinical research to explore the effectiveness, safety and acceptability of medical abortion (Coyaji et al., 2001; 2002; Elul, Ellertson and Winikoff, 1999; Winikoff et al., 1997), limited research has been carried out on issues such as women's experiences of this new method, availability, affordability and providers' perspectives, although some studies are currently under way.

Sex-selective abortion

With the introduction of amniocentesis to detect abnormalities of the foetus, sex determination techniques have been available in India since 1975. The expansion of facilities offering sonography in the mid-1980s made testing for sex determination widely and easily available. Although the government has tried to curb the increase in sex-selective abortions by introducing the PNDT Act in 1994, the Act proved to be ineffective in preventing such abortions (Oomman and Ganatra, 2002). This is not surprising given the strong son preference prevailing in most parts of the country, the loopholes in the Act per se and in its enforcement.

Recent evidence, both direct and indirect, highlight that the number of sex-selective abortions has increased vastly (Oomman and Ganatra, 2002). This is indirectly reflected in the latest Census figures which indicate that the child (0-6 years) sex ratio has declined from 945 females per 1,000 males in 1991 to 927 females per 1,000 males in 2001 (RGI, 2001). Although it is difficult to quantify precisely the prevalence/incidence of sex-selective abortion, a growing number of community- and facility-based studies provide direct and indirect estimates. A number of community-based studies in different parts of the country report a prevalence of sex-selective abortion ranging from 3-17 per cent over different reference periods, i.e., two years preceding the survey to life-time (Elul et al., 2003; Malhotra et al., 2003; Ganatra, Hirve and Rao, 2000; Khanna, 1997).

Facility-based studies report a much higher prevalence; for example, two in five women with one or more daughters, but no living sons had had an abortion in a Patiala hospital (Sahi and Sarin, 1996). Indirect estimates derived from NFHS 2 data indicate that among women who received ultrasound or amniocentesis during antenatal check-ups, 6.4 per cent of the female foetuses can be assumed to have been aborted (Arnold, Kishor and Roy, 2002).

Available evidence shows that the practice of sex-selective abortion cuts across all socio-economic groups (Booth, Verma and Beri, 1994; Ganatra, Hirve and Rao, 2000; George and Dahiya, 1998). In several studies, sex-selective abortion is reported to be a family building strategy to achieve the conflicting goals of limiting family size and achieving the desired sex composition (Ganatra, 2000). For example, the prevalence of sex-selective abortion is found to be higher among women with one or more living daughters but no living sons (Booth, Verma and Beri, 1994). However, some studies report that sex-selective abortion is practised by couples who already have a living son or no children (Ganatra, Hirve and Rao, 2000; George and Dahiya, 1998). Further, evidence from qualitative studies indicates that sex-selective abortion is perceived and projected as an easy alternative to female infanticide, a way to save girl children from an unhappy life and a means to prevent dowry payment in future (Khanna, 1997; Verma, Bracken and Elul, 2003): "To give birth to a female child would mean spoiling her life as well as her parent's life. So, we felt it was right to abort the female foetus" (27-year-old woman with a son and a daughter; Verma, Bracken and Elul, 2003).

While sex-selective abortion per se is little researched, decision-making related to sex-selective abortion is even less explored. Limited evidence available from a small-scale qualitative study, though not generalisable, reports that the decision to pursue a sex-selective abortion is taken primarily by the couple; at the same time, providers appear to play a key role in providing information on sex-determination services: "Either you get your abortion before sonography or after, I will charge you the same money but if God hears your wish and the foetus is found to be male, then you can escape from abortion." (41-year-old woman with four daughters narrating her experiences with a provider; Verma, Bracken and Elul, 2003).

Magnitude and context

Official figures report that about 0.6 million induced abortions take place annually in India (Khan et al., 1999). Given that only approximately 10 per cent of abortions are conducted by qualified providers in approved institutions (Khan, Barge and Philip, 1996), and that abortions taking place at registered facilities are grossly under-reported (Chhabra and Nuna, 1994; Ganatra, 2000; Khan et al., 1999), this represents only a fraction of the total number of induced abortions taking place in the country. Indirect estimates for the year 1991, using parameters arrived at on the basis of a small-scale study conducted in 1966, project the number of induced abortions annually at 6.7 million (Chhabra and Nuna, 1994).

Estimates of the prevalence of induced abortion derived from community-based surveys, again likely to be grossly underestimated as women tend to under-report the incidence of induced abortions in survey settings, show wide variations. For example, NFHS 2 data reveal that 1.7 per cent of all pregnancies over a lifetime ended in induced abortions (IIPS and ORC Macro, 2000). In comparison, small-scale studies report 3.4-14.0 induced abortions per 100 live births (Ganatra, 2000; Malhotra et al., 2003).

Profile of abortion seekers

While women of all age groups seek abortion in India, a recent review suggests that the majority of those seeking abortion are 20-29 years (Ganatra, 2000). A substantial number of adolescents, both married and unmarried, also seek abortion services. Between 1-10 per cent of abortion seekers are adolescents (Ganatra, 2000), though a few facility-based studies report that the proportion of adolescent abortion seekers is as high as one in three (Chhabra et al., 1988; Solapurkar and Sangam, 1985). Nationally, data from NFHS 1998-99 show a lifetime induced abortion ratio of 1.1 among married adolescents (Pachauri and Santhya, 2002b).

The vast majority of women seeking abortion in India are married, though about 2-30 per cent are unmarried (Ganatra, 2000). Among the unmarried, adolescents constitute a disproportionately large percentage of those who seek abortion. At least one-half of unmarried women seeking abortions are adolescents, many of whom are below 15 years (Jejeebhoy, 1996).

Reasons for seeking abortion

Although official records show that contraceptive failure and risk to mother's health are leading reasons for women seeking abortion (Chhabra and Nuna, 1994; Sood, Juneja and Goyal, 1995), studies suggest a different picture. Several studies indicate that most abortions are sought to limit family size or space the next pregnancy (Elul et al., 2003; Ganatra, 2000; Malhotra et al., 2003). For example, in a study in Madhya Pradesh, women reported achievement of desired family size as the reason in 41 per cent of attempted abortions, and the need for spacing in 30 per cent of abortion attempts (Malhotra et al., 2003). A few recent studies indicate that risk to women's health is also a relatively common reason for seeking abortion (Elul et al., 2003; Malhotra et al., 2003). For example, a study in Madhya Pradesh found that women reported health reasons in 22 per cent of attempted abortions (Malhotra et al., 2003).

Less commonly reported reasons for seeking abortion include contraceptive failure, pregnancies occurring soon after marriage or occurring outside of marriage or problems with the foetus (Ganatra, 2000; Malhotra et al., 2003). For example, a review shows that only a small proportion of women seeking abortion (fewer than 5 per cent) reported contraceptive failure as the reason for an abortion (Ganatra, 2000). Even though first pregnancy is highly valued and hence women generally do not opt for induced abortion, a study in Madhya Pradesh shows that women mentioned a pregnancy that happened too soon after marriage in 6 per cent of abortion attempts (Malhotra et al., 2003).

Type of provider

Available evidence, though limited, indicates that the majority of abortions take place in private facilities (Ganatra, Hirve and Rao, 2000; ICMR, 1989; Malhotra et al., 2003; Ramachandar, 2002). For example, in a community-based study in Madhya Pradesh, more than one-half of abortions among urban women took place in a private facility compared to one-fourth of abortions in a public sector facility and the remaining resorting to folk methods or self-induction (Malhotra et al., 2003). However, a study in Rajasthan indicates that one-half of the women sought abortion from a public sector provider (Elul et al., 2003), though it is not clear whether the service was dispensed in a public or a private sector facility.

The practice of self-induction or using lay practitioners is declining among abortion seekers in general, though adolescents, unmarried women, rural and economically disadvantaged women still rely on [these methods (Ganatra, 2000; Gupte, Bandewar and Pisal, 1996; Malhotra et al., 2003). For example, in a study in Madhya Pradesh, 56 per cent of rural women relied on folk methods or self-induction (Malhotra et al., 2003).

Mortality and morbidity

There is limited information on abortion-related maternal deaths in India (Johnston, 2002). A conservative estimate places the number of abortion-related deaths in a year in India at 15,000-20,000 (Chhabra and Nuna, 1994). Official figures indicate that unsafe abortion accounted for 9 per cent of maternal deaths in the year 1998 (RGI, 2000). However, evidence from facility-based studies suggests that abortion-related complications account for 2.5-30 per cent of maternal deaths taking place in hospitals (Ganatra, 2000).

Abortion-related mortality represents only a fraction of abortion-related complications, and many more women experience life-threatening and other morbidities. For example, in a community-based study in Madhya Pradesh, more than one in two abortion attempts among rural women (57 per cent) and more than two in five abortion attempts among urban women (46 per cent) resulted in at least one complication. The complications were severe in one-third of abortion attempts among rural women and one-sixth of attempts among urban women (Malhotra et al., 2003). The most frequently reported abortion-related morbidities are menstrual irregularities, backache, and excessive bleeding (Elul et al., 2003; Ganatra, 2000). Little data exist on chronic abortion-related morbidities, including pelvic inflammatory disease, secondary infertility and the risk of future ectopic pregnancy (Ganatra, 2000).

As is widely recognised, abortion-related complications are higher when performed by inadequately trained providers or in unhygienic conditions. For example, a study in West Bengal reports a complication rate of 12.2 per cent for abortions conducted by a specialist, 45.8 per cent by a private general practitioner, and 100 per cent by unqualified providers or paramedics (Mondal, 1991). Similarly, second trimester abortions carry a higher risk of complications (Bhathena, Sheriar and Guillebaud, 1990; Ganatra, 2000; Johnston, 2002). A hospital-based study reveals that the risk of abortion complications is 12 times higher for second trimester abortions than first trimester ones (ICMR, 1989). Unmarried adolescents, women who are illiterate and those living in rural areas are perhaps more prone to major abortion complications because they seek late abortions or use the services of unqualified abortion providers (Ganatra, 2000; Jejeebhoy, 1996; Johnston, 2002; Malhotra et al., 2003).

Factors underlying persistence of unsafe abortions

Despite the liberalisation of abortion services and the introduction of safer abortion techniques, abortion continues to be unsafe for the vast majority of women seeking such services. Several factors operating at the individual, family, and community level contribute to this situation, some of which are discussed below.

Lack of awareness

Lack of awareness of the legal status of abortion and the facilities where abortion services are legally provided may lead many women to seek abortion from untrained and unqualified providers. Studies in different parts of the country show that even though abortion has been legalised in India for more than three decades, only a small minority of men and women know that abortion is legal (Elul et al., 2003; ICMR, 1989; Khan, Barge and Philip, 1996; Malhotra et al., 2003). For example, in a community-based study in Rajasthan, only one in six men and women were aware that abortion is legal. Even more alarming was that nearly four in five men and more than one in two women believed it is illegal (Elul et al., 2003), and formal services are less likely to be sought when women perceive abortion to be illegal (Ganatra, 2000). Even when women are aware of the legal status of abortion, they may not be fully aware of the conditions under which abortion is allowed. For example, in a study in Madhya Pradesh, while 15 per cent of women knew that abortion is legal, only 9 per cent knew the correct timing under which abortion is legally permitted (Malhotra et al., 2003). Misconceptions about the conditions under which abortion services are provided are common; for example, husband's consent is needed for seeking abortion (Elul et al., 2003; Gupte, Bandewar and Pisal, 1997). Moreover, often women may not be aware of the existence of registered facilities where these services can be accessed (ICMR, 1989; Mukhopadhyay and Garimella, 1998).

Apart from lack of awareness of the legal status of abortion and registered facilities, lack of awareness about pregnancy may contribute to many women, especially adolescent girls, delaying seeking abortion services and obtaining care from unqualified providers (Jejeebhoy, 2000a).

Limited access to services

Although the number of approved abortion facilities in India has increased significantly from 1,877 in 1972-76 to 9,467 in 1997 (Khan et al., 1999), access to safe abortion services continues to be limited for the vast majority of women in the country. In fact, some of the clauses in the MTP Act, 1972 have in effect contributed to restricting the availability and access to abortion services (Khan et al., 1999). For example, only gynaecologists or physician who have received training in MTP are allowed to perform an abortion, and only in government clinics or hospitals, or institutions approved by the government for this purpose. Moreover, the approval of two doctors is required to abort pregnancies between 12 and 20 weeks' gestation. Stringent criteria for the approval of centres, although well intentioned, have in effect restricted the expansion of registered facilities in the private and non-governmental sectors (Barua, 2002; Iyengar and Iyengar, 2002; Sheriar, 2001). The decentralisation of authority for the approval of MTP centres and the government's commitment to increase access to abortion services at the primary health care level may improve the availability of abortion facilities in the near future (GOI, 2002; Mallik, 2002).

Not only are the approved facilities inadequate in number, but they are also distributed unevenly between and within states. For example, Maharashtra with 10 per cent of India's population has more than one-fifth of the total number of facilities in the country. In contrast, Bihar, also with about 10 per cent of the total population, has only 1 per cent of the facilities (Khan et al., 1999). Within each state, the approved facilities are concentrated in urban areas, resulting in limited access for a vast majority of women in rural areas (Chhabra and Nuna, 1994; Khan, Barge and Philip, 1996).

Even where approved facilities exist, services in the public sector are rarely or erratically provided due to the lack of trained manpower or equipment or both (Khan et al., 1998; 1999). For example, district-level teaching institutions, sub-district hospitals, community health centres, postpartum centres and primary health centres are required to provide abortion services. However, a situation analysis of abortion facilities in Gujarat, Maharashtra, Uttar Pradesh and Tamil Nadu shows that only about one-fourth to nearly three-fifths of the primary health centres offered abortion services (Khan et al., 1999). The most recently conducted national level facility survey reports that only 3 per cent of the primary health centres provide MTP services. The survey also reports that most primary health centres lack essential equipment. Only one in six primary health centres, for example, have MTP suction aspirators (IIPS, 2001a).

Poor quality of services

Few studies have explored the quality of abortion services in the public and private sector, particularly in the private sector. Available evidence highlights the poor quality of abortion services.

Often providers in the public and private sector are not trained or are inadequately trained (Barge, 2002; Barua, 2002; Khan et al., 1999). The most recently conducted national level facility survey reports that only 13 per cent of primary health centres in the country have at least one medical officer trained in MTP. The situation is worse in several states including Bihar, Haryana, Madhya Pradesh, Rajasthan, Uttar Pradesh and West Bengal where only 2-6 per cent of primary health centres have a medical officer trained in providing MTP services (IIPS, 2001a). In a facility study in Haryana, nearly one-third of the 52 private providers had not received any training on conducting an abortion. Similarly, in Maharashtra, more than one-third of the public sector providers and more than two-fifths of the private sector providers were reported to be untrained (Barge, 2002). Moreover, as there are few MTP cases in the training centres, trainee doctors do not receive sufficient practical experience in conducting MTPs so even after training many providers do not feel competent to provide services (Khan et al., 1999). Further, it is reported that most teaching hospitals prefer to offer training on electric vacuum aspiration, dilation and curettage and induction methods rather than manual vacuum aspiration, a relatively simple method of abortion (Barge et al., 1997; Khan et al., 1998; 1999).

The judgemental attitude of providers in public and private sector facilities, particularly in the public sector, is likely to force many women to seek informal sector providers who are unlikely to provide safe services: "in the government hospital the nurses demand money and also use abusive language. In X's nursing home, the doctor does not use bad language. We can get an abortion and sterilisation done on the same day and return to our house. Hospitalisation is just for one day. The waiting time is only one hour. Things are fast and if we have any problems we can go back to him" (Ramachandar, 2002). Studies show that providers often disregard the need to respect the privacy and confidentiality of women seeking abortion: "privacy and confidentiality is not an issue with women. After all where can you get more anonymity than at a public hospital where thousands are milling around in the out-patient department?" (Barua, 2002). Coercive contraception following an MTP is not uncommon, and many women reportedly refuse to go to a primary health care centre for an MTP because they do not want to get sterilised (Barge et al., 1998; Gupta, 1993; Gupte, Bandewar and Pisal, 1997; Ramachandar, 2002). Further, several studies highlight that providers often insist on husband's consent, though the law does not mandate it nor is it preferred by women (Elul et al., 2003; Ganatra, 2000; Gupte, Bandewar and Pisal, 1999). In a study in Rajasthan, four in five women reported that the provider took their husband's consent (Elul et al., 2003). Moreover, even when services exist, providers may selectively refuse services to some women. For example, a study in Maharashtra reports that 40 per cent of providers selectively refused services to unmarried and separated young women, of whom 24 per cent were in legally recognised MTP centres (Ganatra, 2002b).

Studies show that pre- and post-abortion services have often been given a low priority. For example, a study among abortion service providers in slums in Gujarat reports that no physical or internal check-ups were carried out, and only cursory enquiries about medical and obstetric history were taken (Barua, 2002). Moreover, women were not often informed of the possible risks of the procedure, potential complications and their treatment, need for a follow-up visit, and post-abortion contraception, especially the range of contraceptive choices available to prevent repeat abortions (Barge et al., 1998; Barua, 2002; Khan et al., 1999; Prakasamma, 2002). A multi-state study reports that less than one-half of women were informed about the possibility of infection (Khan et al., 1999). A study in Andhra Pradesh indicates that follow-up care was provided only in selected cases by auxiliary nurse midwives (Prakasamma, 2002). Moreover, emergency services to deal with incomplete abortion and life threatening post-abortion complications are totally lacking in the current service delivery system (Johnston, 2002).

Cost of services

Even though there is evidence that women are willing to pay for services that meet their needs and perceptions of quality (Ganatra, Hirve and Rao, 2000), the financial burden of abortion services is substantial (Gupte, Bandewar and Pisal, 1997; Maitra, 1998). Economic constraints may compel many women, particularly those who are poor and dependent on others, to seek services from unqualified providers (Elul et al., 2003; Kerrigan, Gaffikin and Magarick, 1995; Malhotra et al., 2003; Parivar Seva Sanstha, 1998). Unfortunately, in public sector facilities that are expected to provide services free of cost, it is reported that women incur hidden costs in the form of cost of medicine and illegal fees for staff (Barge, Manjunath and Nair, 1994; Barge et al., 1997, 1998; Chhabra and Nuna, 1994; ICMR, 1989; Kerrigan, Gaffikin and Magarick, 1995; Khan et al., 1999). A study in Madhya Pradesh reports that only one in ten abortions in public sector MTP centres were provided free of cost (Malhotra et al., 2003).

Gender roles and norms

Available evidence, though limited, reveals that gender roles and norms operate in many ways to limit women's access to safe services. Even though a number of studies report that the decision to undergo an abortion among married women is taken jointly by the woman and her husband (Elul et al., 2003; Ganatra, Hirve and Rao, 2000; Malhotra et al., 2003; Sinha et al., 1998), a not-so insignificant proportion of women, especially unmarried and married young women, may find it difficult to take decisions on their own regarding abortion or to communicate about abortion-related needs to those who wield power in the household (Barua and Kurz, 2001; Malhotra et al., 2003), leading to delays in seeking abortion and thereby jeopardising safety. For example, in a community-based study in Madhya Pradesh, husbands, unilaterally or jointly, played the major decision-making role in 20 per cent of abortion attempts (Malhotra et al., 2003). Moreover, studies show that some women who wish to terminate a pregnancy may face opposition from the family (Ganatra, 2000).

Stigma attached to abortion, particularly when sought by women who are not currently married, may also compel women to delay seeking services or to seek services from confidential but unsafe providers (Ganatra and Hirve, 2002a). For example, in a study in Pune, women seeking an abortion outside of marriage ranked confidentiality, discreetness and distant location of abortion services as the most important indicators of quality of services (Gupte, Bandewar and Pisal, 1999). Yet another study in Pune reports that nearly one-fourth of unmarried women sought abortion services from traditional providers compared to 2 per cent of married women (Ganatra, Hirve and Rao, 2000).

Finally, the increasing practice of sex-selective abortion also tends to place women at risk of undergoing unsafe abortion. Women attempting sex-selective abortions may not opt for legal abortion services. Sonography can detect foetal sex only at the beginning of the second trimester when the risk of abortion complications is much higher (Bhathena, Sheriar and Guillebaud, 1990; Ganatra, 2000; ICMR, 1989; Johnston, 2002), therefore sex-selective abortion seekers are vulnerable to unsafe abortions.

The way forward

Although abortion services in India were liberalised more than three decades ago, the vast majority of women continue to seek and receive abortion services from unqualified providers. As a result, many women die or suffer serious life-threatening complications. A host of factors notably lack of awareness of the legality of abortion services, limited access to safe services, poor quality of services and gender roles and norms lead women to seek services from untrained providers. In the Indian context, where the preference for sons is particularly strong, the practice of second-trimester sex-selective abortions is becoming widespread.

The introduction of new technologies and legislation is expected to make safe abortion services more accessible. However, the challenge remains in effectively implementing these measures.

Programme recommendations

- The widespread lack of awareness of the legal status of abortion services and women's rights under the existing law as well as of the facilities that offer abortion services call for socially and culturally appropriate IEC campaigns. There is also a strong need for efforts to promote awareness of the dangers of unsafe abortion practices and the gestational age at which safe abortion can be obtained. Equally important are communication efforts to remove stigma associated with induced abortion.
- Given the uneven distribution of existing facilities, efforts to increase accessibility of safe abortion services to hitherto unserved or under-served areas and population groups, including adolescents, need to be vigorously pursued. The lack of trained manpower needs to be addressed by improving training facilities and facilitating the training of private practitioners. The training curriculum should include new and safer methods of abortion, including manual vacuum aspiration techniques and medical abortion, as well as emphasise quality of care elements.
- Given the poor quality of existing abortion services in the country, establishing service delivery guidelines regarding technical standards of service, patient-provider interaction, confidentiality, pre- and post-abortion counselling and care is critically needed. All existing MTP facilities should be regularly monitored and evaluated.

Research recommendations

- Research on abortion has increased in recent years, but significant gaps in our understanding of the multiple dimensions of abortion seeking behaviour prevail. Evidence on the prevalence and patterns of abortion is limited, and even the latest available estimate of induced abortion is more than a decade old. The need for assessing the incidence of induced abortion, using multiple and innovative methods of data collection cannot be over-emphasised.

- Abortion-related needs and service seeking patterns of many vulnerable groups including adolescents, unmarried, divorced or separated women remain less studied and hence there is need for future studies to focus on these sub-population groups.
- The review highlights that the practice of sex-selective abortion is increasingly becoming common in many parts of the country. An in-depth understanding of the prevalence/incidence and perspectives of those involved in decisions on sex-selective abortion, clients' profile and experiences is needed to formulate effective policies and programmes to prevent this practice.
- Very little information exists on abortion-related complications, especially chronic complications. Follow-up studies are needed to estimate the extent of these complications and their implications for women's health and well being.
- There is a need to explore the potential of paramedics to conduct early abortion and provide abortion related care through well-designed studies.
- Studies show that the quality of abortion services in the country is generally poor. The constraints that providers face in providing quality service need to be explored to design more appropriate interventions.
- While abortion per se is less studied, the pathways between pregnancy and abortion are even less explored in India. An in-depth understanding of the complex nature of abortion-related decision-making, provider choice and the actual utilisation of abortion services would help in designing effective interventions to improve access to services.

Infertility

Anjali Widge

Though the ICPD Programme of Action states that reproductive health services should include the prevention and appropriate treatment of infertility (United Nations, 1994), there is inadequate focus on infertility in India's reproductive health programme. Yet the number of infertile persons remains significant, particularly in the Indian social and cultural context, and the impact on women's lives is considerable. Care-seeking options continue to be few and services available in the public sector are inadequate.

The difficulties of measuring infertility are compounded by its multiple definitions. The World Health Organisation (WHO), using a two-year reference period, defines primary infertility as the lack of conception despite cohabitation and exposure to pregnancy (WHO, 1991). Some studies use childlessness as a definition (women with no live birth) based on various reference periods, ranging from one to five years, making comparison difficult. Secondary infertility is defined as the failure to conceive following a previous pregnancy despite cohabitation and exposure to pregnancy (in the absence of contraception, breastfeeding or postpartum amenorrhoea) (WHO, 1991).

There is little evidence on the levels and patterns of infertility in India. According to studies conducted by WHO, the extent of primary and secondary infertility in India is 3 and 8 per cent respectively. Recent NFHS 2 data, using childlessness as an indicator, estimates that 3.8 per cent of currently married women between the ages of 40-49 are childless. Based on 1981 Census data, childlessness amongst ever-married women in India is estimated to be about 6 per cent (Vermuri and Manohar, 1986). Evidence from community-based studies from across India suggests similar prevalence rates for childlessness (Bang et al., 1989; Kanani, Latha and Shah, 1994; Mulgaonkar, 2001; Unisa, 1999).

Although the consequences for women's lives and the health-seeking behaviour of women with primary and secondary infertility could be different, most population-based studies in India have not explored these issues separately. Therefore, this review does not make such a distinction.

The causes of primary and secondary infertility relate to both males and females, and the conditions that directly contribute to infertility vary widely by region and culture (Farley and Belsey, 1988). According to WHO multi-centric studies of infertility in India, 40 per cent of women and 73 per cent of men had no demonstrable cause of infertility (Cates, Farely and Rowe, 1985a). Tubal factor was the most common cause of infertility among women (nearly 30 per cent), followed by anovulation (22 per cent). Among men, accessory gland infection was the most common factor for infertility (8.8 per cent) (Cates, Farely and Rowe, 1985b).

In cases where infertility is caused by infections, leading underlying factors are STIs (Farley and Belsey, 1988) and iatrogenic factors, including unsafe abortions and unhygienic delivery conditions (Kochar, 1980). The WHO study shows, for example, that the dominant cause of infertility in Asia among women with a demonstrable cause was on account of either an STI or unsafe management of abortion or delivery. Among men with a demonstrable cause, about one in three may have become infertile as a result of an STI experience (Cates, Farely and Rowe, 1985b). In India, the prevalence of STIs was found to be high among women reporting infertility and pelvic inflammatory disease (Bhujwala et al., 1988; Brabin et al., 1998; Chhabra and Fali, 1992; Kushtagi et al., 1991).

Socio-cultural context and consequences

In a patriarchal setting, such as in India, bearing children, particularly sons, largely defines a woman's identity. Motherhood is of great social significance and infertility is perceived as a threat to men's procreativity and the continuity of the lineage (Iyengar and Iyengar, 1999; Jindal and Dhall, 1990; Jindal and Gupta, 1989; Mulgaonkar 2001; Neff, 1994; Patel, 1994; Prakasamma, 1999b; Singh and Dhaliwal, 1993; Unisa, 1999; Widge, 2001).

Infertility is a life crisis with invisible losses, and its consequences are manifold. Childless women experience stigma and isolation. Infertility can threaten a woman's identity, status and economic security and consequently, be a major source of anxiety leading to lowered self-esteem and a sense of powerlessness. Although perceptions of women's roles and attitudes may be shifting, particularly in the upper and middle classes, bearing a child still remains an important factor in the socio-economic well being of most Indian women (Das Gupta, Chen and Krishnan, 1995).

Infertility can also result in a strained relationship in the marital home. Men tend to hold their wives responsible for infertility and many wives tend to blame themselves for childlessness irrespective of who may be responsible (Desai, Shrinivasan and Hazra, 1992). In some cases women are threatened with another marriage or divorce and many fear abandonment and loss of social and economic security. They could also be victims of violence, abuse and social exclusion (Singh, Dhaliwal and Kaur, 1996). Some couples experience altered sexual responses (Desai, Shrinivasan and Hazra, 1992; Mulgaonkar, 2001). Though childlessness usually has a negative impact on marriage, some husbands are supportive and defend their wives against family pressure or criticism (Widge, 2001).

Treatment-seeking

Women go through various treatment-seeking modes to avoid the adverse consequences of childlessness. Adoption is not an acceptable option for many as women face psychological, familial and community pressure to produce a biological child (Iyengar and Iyengar, 1999; Singh and Dhaliwal, 1993; Unisa, 1999). Couples seek varied traditional methods and religious practices, including visits to temples, abstaining from visiting a place where a woman has delivered a child, observing *tantric* rites, wearing charms, participating in rituals and visiting astrologers (Desai, Shrinivasan and Hazra, 1992; Patel, 1994; Unisa, 1999).

A variety of treatments are sought though a pattern of treatment-seeking does not clearly emerge. Some studies suggest that women first seek treatment from traditional healers (Gupta, Dhall and Dhaliwal, 1983; Kakar, 1983). More recent studies have identified allopathy as the first treatment sought. Couples also follow religious practices with such treatment, either simultaneously or subsequently (Mulgaonkar, 2001; Unisa, 1999). As a last resort, when allopathic treatment does not work, women seek other methods, such as *ayurveda*, homeopathy, *unani* and other traditional methods, or visit holy places and spiritual healers (Unisa, 1999).

Most couples seek treatment after trying to conceive for one to four years (Gupta, Dhall and Dhaliwal, 1983; Iyengar and Iyengar, 1999; Mulgaonkar, 2001; Unisa, 1999). Couples may delay seeking medical advice because of the fear of a final definite diagnosis, emotional stress, the physical discomfort of the tests they would have to undergo and admitting failure in their efforts to conceive (Gupta, Dhall and Dhaliwal, 1983). Irrespective of who the infertile person is, it is the woman who usually initiates the first contact with a physician (Gupta, Dhall and Dhaliwal, 1983). Couples with primary infertility are usually more interested in treatment than those with secondary infertility (Gupta, Dhall and Dhaliwal, 1983; Singh, Dhaliwal and Kaur, 1996). Treatment sometimes continues over a long period; for example, in one study, women sought allopathic treatment for 25 years and some continued to rely on rituals or religious practices for over 30 years (Unisa, 1999). Although most studies reveal that male participation in infertility diagnosis and treatment tends to be limited as infertility is perceived to be a woman's problem, in some contexts, husbands also participate and accept treatment if required (Unisa, 1999).

Stigmatising beliefs, limited male participation, cost, indifferent quality of care and lack of services in the public sector are major barriers to prompt and appropriate treatment-seeking. Patterns of treatment-seeking depend on the woman/couple's socio-economic status, decision-making within the family, the level of information and accessibility of treatment (Iyengar and Iyengar, 1999; Singh, Dhaliwal and Kaur, 1996; Unisa, 1999). High costs sometimes results in discontinuation of treatment or resort to unqualified practitioners (Singh, Dhaliwal and Kaur, 1996). Traditional beliefs about women being possessed by evil spirits also inhibit women from seeking appropriate treatment (Iyengar and Iyengar, 1999).

The public health system does not offer access to adequate preventive, curative and counselling services. Though infertility treatment is theoretically available at government facilities, effective treatment is often difficult to access as there is little coordination between gynaecologists, infertility specialists, surgeons and laboratory technicians. Services are available in the private sector but are of varying quality and costs.

Seeking assisted reproductive technologies

There is now an increasing trend towards using ARTs, such as artificial insemination by husband/donor, *in vitro* fertilisation (IVF), gamete intra-fallopian transfer and intra cytoplasmic sperm injection. Such advanced technologies are generally pursued only as a last resort after less intrusive alternatives have been exhausted (Widge, 2001). However, there has recently been an increase in the demand for artificial insemination, possibly because it is perceived to increase the chances of having a male child through sex-selection methods (Gupta, 2000). In some contexts there seems to be low acceptance of artificial insemination by a donor among couples (Jindal and Gupta, 1989; Mulgaonkar, 2001).

Although ARTs offer hope to the infertile to bear a biological child, a number of issues remain to be addressed. ART services are not usually available at public health facilities but are increasingly being offered in private clinics. As services are expensive and highly commercialised, the high costs of ART treatment tends to create a situation of exploitation of childless couples and exacerbates their vulnerability, which has deterred many couples from seeking such services. Couples often do not have easy access to information on ARTs and select doctors through trial and error. Even when these services are accessed, they provide inadequate information and counselling. Informed consent procedures are also generally unsatisfactory.

A major concern in the present context of ART services in India is with regard to the quality of care. Services are not regulated and the quality of treatment is variable, ranging from clinics that offer professional and high quality services to those that are run by unqualified practitioners. Unscrupulous providers may encourage the repeated use of these technologies, and women may have to endure many cycles of testing, experimentation and treatment. ARTs like IVF are experienced to be physiologically, emotionally and financially stressful (Widge, 2001).

The success rate of such technologies remains unclear. The Indian Council of Medical Research reports an average take-home baby rate of 20-30 per cent per IVF cycle (ICMR, 2000), but this estimate has not been substantiated by any studies. Leading clinics in India claim a 30-40 per cent success rate (which is usually the pregnancy rate) but it may be considerably lower (Gupta, 2000; Widge, 2001).

Inadequate monitoring and regulation of such services is leading to the misuse of these technologies, including IVF-related sex pre-selection methods, and the proliferation of unethical practices. Ethical issues such as the manipulation of sperms, eggs and embryos, the commercialisation of technology, and the wider implications of surrogacy/commercial surrogacy need to be addressed through effective regulatory mechanisms. The Indian Council of Medical Research has recently drafted national guidelines for the regulation of ART clinics, but it remains to be seen how these are implemented (ICMR, 2002).

The policy context

Government policies in India have largely ignored the issue of infertility. The National Population Policy, 2000 mentions it only briefly in the context of providing information, counselling and regular supply of medication *only* for communities like tribals, and displaced and migrant populations who 'may not need fertility regulation' (MOHFW, 2000). There is also limited focus on services for the infertile in the Reproductive and Child Health Programme. Though the Tenth Five-year Plan (2002-07) has discussed access to essential clinical examination, investigation, management and counselling services for infertility, such services are in practice rarely available in the public sector.

The way forward

In patriarchal settings such as India where a woman's identity is determined by her ability to bear children, particularly sons, infertility can have far-reaching consequences. Women tend to seek care from a variety of providers, including unqualified practitioners, further increasing their vulnerability. The availability of new technologies, such as ARTs, offers hope to infertile couples, but there is growing concern about its misuse, particularly in the absence of adequate information and counselling and appropriate mechanisms for regulation.

Prevention and treatment of infertility is possible in low resource settings, and reproductive health programmes can be an entry point for couples with infertility problems. However, there is a need to enhance existing services and improve the quality of care for infertile couples.

Programme recommendations

- Services for infertility treatment should be integrated into the larger reproductive and child health package of services. A policy on infertility care as part of an integrated reproductive health care programme could be formulated based on an analysis and evaluation of the functioning of the actual health care infrastructure and its availability and effectiveness. Investigations for infertility could be conducted at various levels of the health care system. For instance, service provision at the subcentre/urban health post level could include couple counselling on fertility-related issues and appropriate referral for STIs. Basic diagnostic tests, treatment of some STIs and referral services could be provided at the primary health centre and rural hospital level, while specialised tests and advanced treatment could be provided at the tertiary level.
- Health care providers at each level need to be trained to impart screening, examination, diagnosis, referral and treatment services as appropriate.
- Information should be provided on the preventive and curative aspects of infertility treatment, and appropriate and effective information campaigns designed to encourage preventive practices, and reduce the stigmatisation and social exclusion of infertile women and men. Information on adoption should be made available.
- Effective mechanisms need to be implemented to regulate and manage high technology treatments for infertility (such as ARTs), which are offered mostly in the private sector, have low success rates and are expensive. Guidelines should be implemented in a manner that doctors are compelled to look critically at issues of informed consent, screening donors, legal and ethical issues and quality of care. Policies should ensure that the rights of women as users of these technologies are not in any way compromised. The issue of exploitation of patients in low-resource settings should be addressed.

Research recommendations

- Few studies have explored the service delivery setting and identified gaps in services. Documenting these issues would be an important step in addressing infertility in a public health context and providing programmatic inputs.
- It has been argued that infertility treatment is not cost-effective. Research on operationally feasible and cost-effective treatment on infertility in low-resource settings is required to make such treatment widely available.
- There is a paucity of data on the perceptions and experiences of infertility. Community-based studies that explore the socio-cultural dimensions of infertility, men's attitudes towards infertility, the stigma associated with infertility, existing support systems or lack of them, mechanisms to bring about change and attitudes and barriers to adoption could contribute substantially to understanding the context of infertility.
- Women's experiences with ARTs need to be explored as there is a paucity of data on this subject.

Reproductive Tract and Sexually Transmitted Infections

K.G. Santhya

The prevention and control of RTIs and STIs, including HIV, have become a national priority. Research and programmatic efforts have been significantly enhanced over the last decade, however, the epidemic continues to spread widely and remains a public health as well as a development challenge.

Prevalence

It is difficult to estimate precisely the prevalence of RTIs/STIs in the Indian context. Current surveillance systems for STIs/HIV do not provide a complete picture of the incidence of these infections or trends over time. Moreover, data from population-based and facility- or convenience-based studies are variable and cannot be compared as different sampling methods, laboratory procedures and criteria are used for diagnosis (Hawkes and Santhya, 2001; Oomman, 2000).

In the early 1990s, the annual incidence of STIs was estimated at around 5 per cent of the adult population, which implies that about 40 million new STI cases are occurring annually in the

Insights provided by H. Grosskurth and G. Rangaiyan are gratefully acknowledged.

country (NACO, 1998). This is possibly a conservative estimate of the actual number of cases as it is based on surveillance data from public sector STD clinics, which are mainly located in urban areas and utilised by only 5-10 per cent of patients with STIs (NACO, 1998).

Reported prevalence rates of bacterial, protozoal and viral infections among men and women in facility- and community-based studies are reflected in Tables 5 and 6. Figures reveal that the prevalence of RTIs/STIs is high not only among high-risk population groups but also among low-risk groups in many parts of the country, including rural areas. Clinic-based data indicate that genital ulcer diseases, particularly syphilis, predominate among both men and women. Further, the review indicates that the incidence of viral infections is increasing and, in recent years, has grown from around 3 per cent to nearly a fourth of all infections seen at sexually transmitted disease (STD) clinics, in some cases outstripping rates of bacterial infection (Kumar et al., 2002; Ramasubban, 2000).

In 2002, between 3.82-4.58 million adults in India were estimated to be living with HIV (NACO, 2003a). As of November 2003, a total of 57,781 people in India have been diagnosed with AIDS (NACO, 2003a). Most of these infections have been acquired through sexual transmission (both heterosexual and homosexual) (85 per cent). A smaller number (3 per cent each) have been infected through injecting drug use, infected blood transfusion and mother to child transmission (NACO, 2003a). The infection has now spread from urban to rural areas and from high-risk population groups to the general population. India does not have a single HIV epidemic, but has multiple epidemics in different geographical settings and among different people with different type of risk. Significant variations among and within states are also observed. For example, currently the prevalence (as indicated by the prevalence among STD clinic patients and antenatal women) is highest in Andhra Pradesh, Tamil Nadu, Karnataka, Maharashtra, Goa and Manipur. Variation within states are also observed, for example, HIV prevalence among STD clinic patients in the state of Maharashtra excluding Mumbai is 7.6 per cent, compared to 14.8 per cent in Mumbai (Bose, 2003).

Table 5

STI rates among men in India

Study population	*Prevalence ranges (%)*								
	GC	*CT*	*Syphilis*	*Chancroid (clinical diagnosis)*	*TV*	*HSV*	*HPV (clinical diagnosis)*	*HbsAg*	*HIV*
Community-based or convenience samples									
15-45 year old men[1]	3.4-3.5	1.1-2.0	0.3	—	—	1.0	—	6.0	1.4-1.5
Participants of a community education program[2]	1.7	15.0	—	—	5.6	—	—	—	0.4
Transport and industrial workers[3]	1.8-7.5	0.5-5.3	0.8-21.9	—	1.0-9.9	—	—	3.0-21.2	1.9-10.9
Facility-based									
STD clinic patients[4]	8.5-25.9	20.0-30.0	12.6-57.0	16.1-34.7	—	3.0-14.9	4.9-14.3	3.6-8.8	2.0-7.4
STD clinic patients with genital ulcers[5]	—	—	—	33.0	—	—	—	—	—
STD clinic patients with urethritis[6]	—	12.0	—	—	—	6.6	—	—	—
Patients attending primary health care[7]	—	—	3.6	—	—	—	—	—	—

Contd...

Contd...

Spouses of females with candida and trichomonas[8]	—	—	—	—	60.6	—	—	—	—
Spouses of females with chlamyida[9]	—	33.3	—	—	—	—	—	—	—

Note: Abbreviations used in Table 5 and 6.
GC= gonorrhoea; CT= *Chlamydia trachomatis*; TV= *Trichomonas vaginalis*; HSV= herpes simplex virus; HPV= human papilloma virus; HbsAg = hepatitis B surface antigen; HIV= human immunodeficiency virus

Sources:
1. APAC, 1998a; Thomas et al., 2002
2. Bang et al., n.d.
3. DFID and FHI, 2001a; 2001b; 2001c; Gawande et al, 2000; Manjunath et al., 2002; Rowley and Berkley, 1998
4. Bhujwala et al., 1984; Chaudhary et al., 1988; Chopra et al., 1990; George et al., 1997; Kamat and Banker, 1993; Kura et al., 1998; Risbud et al., 1999; 2002; Sharma et al., 1989; Singh, Joshi and Bajaj, 1990
5. Kumar, Garg and Baruah, 1990
6. Malathi et al., 2002
7. Rowley and Berkley, 1998
8. Kumar, Garg and Baruah, 1990
9. Mania-Pramanik et al., 2001

Table 6

STI rates among women in India

Study population	*Prevalence ranges (%)*							
	GC	*CT*	*Syphilis*	*TV*	*HSV*	*HPV (clinical diagnosis)*	*HBV*	*HIV*
Community-based								
Ever/currently married women[1]	0.0-4.2	0.5-28.7	0.2-8.8	4.3-27.4	—	11.8	—	—
Unmarried & married women[2]	0.3-3.9	1.4-5.2	0.2-10.5	0.8-14.0	1.4	—	4.8	2.0-2.1
Symptomatic women[3]	—	—	—	16.8	—	—	—	—
Pregnant women[4]	0.3	4.3	1.2-11.0	10.0	—	—	—	—
Facility-based and convenience samples								
STD clinic patients[5]	1.3-20.0	—	29.3-43.3	—	4.0-15.4	6.7-15.6	—	1.2-13.6
Wives of STD patients[6]	2.4	20.3	7.4	3.3	—	—	—	—
Commercial Sex Workers[7]	0.5-19.1	4.6-22.9	4.3-63.0	8.8-54.1	7.5-20.0	0.5	2.0-12.0	2.6-49.9
Gynaecological OPD patients[8]	0.0-5.5	0.2-31.3	4.4-17.0	0.4-26.0	0.3-25.0	0.6-42.4	—	0.0
Antenatal patients[9]	—	2.3	0.9-6.2	17.8	—	—	—	—
Gynaecological patients with vaginitis complaints[10]	0.0-2.6	2.6-20.0	2.2	1.6-17.6	12.0	—	—	—
Gynaecological patients with 'cervical erosion'[11]	—	3.0	—	—	—	—	—	—
Infertility and PID patients[12]	0.1-11.0	0.5-24.2	0.5	0.5	—	—	—	—

Contd...

Contd...

Women with obstetric complications[13]	—	18.8	—	—	—	—	—	—
Acceptors of tubal ligation[14]	0.1-2.2	0.0-0.2	0.5-7.0	0.9	—	—	—	—

Sources:
1. Aggarwal et al., 1999; Bhatia et al., 1997; Chhabra et al., 1991; Garg et al., 2002; Parikh et al., n.d.; Prasad et al., 2000; Santhya, 1999
2. APAC, 1998a, Bang et al., 1989; Oomman, 1996; Thomas et al., 2002
3. Chopra et al., 1990; Kamat and Banker, 1993; Nandan et al., 2001; Singh, Joshi and Bajaj, 1990
4. DFID et al., 2001a; 2001b; 2001c; 2001d; 2001e; 2001f; Mayank, Bahl and Bhandari, 2001
5. Bhatnagar et al., 1991; Chaudhary et al., 1988; Chopra et al., 1990; Gangakhedkar et al., 1997; George et al., 1997; Kamat and Banker, 1993; Mali et al., 1991; Misra et al., 1992; Misra, Das and Chandrawati 2001
6. Divekar et al., 2000; Malathi et al., 2002; Parashari et al., 1994; Singh, Joshi and Bajaj, 1990; Sinha, 1994
7. Divekar et al., 2000; Desai et al., 2003; DFID et al, 2001a; 2001b; 2001c; 2001d; 2001e; 2001f; Gangakhedkar et al., 1997; Jana et al., 1998; Urmil et al., 1989
8. Bhatnagar et al., 1991; Chaudhuri and Iyengar, 1994; Dhall et al., 1990; Gogate et al., 1990; Jayarao et al., 1989; Joshi et al., 1994; Mali et al., 1991; Mishra, Singh and Sharma, 1988; Misra et al., 1992; Misra, Das and Chandravati, 2001; Pal et al., 1993; Parashari et al., 1994; Sinha, 1994; Vajpayee et al., 2000
9. Gupta, Thergaonkar and Chawla, 1998; Hira, 1991; Kunte et al., 1999; Pal et al., 1993; Rowley and Berkley, 1998; Singh et al., 1992; Vajpayee, Seth and Malhotra., 2001
10. Aggarwal et al., 1999; Chhabra et al., 1993; Deb et al., 1989; Kar et al., 1988; Mania-Pramanik et al., 2001; Pandit et al., 1993
11. Chhabra et al., 1993; Kar et al., 1988.
12. Bhujwala et al., 1988; Brabin et al., 1998; Chhabra and Fali, 1992; Kushtagi et al., 1991; Mania-Pramanik et al., 2001; Vishwanath et al., 2000
13. Mania-Pramanik et al., 2001
14. Brabin et al., 1998; Char and Vaidya, 2000

Studies show that the number of cases of women infected within marriage is increasing (Divekar et al., 2000; Gangakhedkar et al., 1997; Mehendale et al., 1996). There is growing evidence that a growing number of women attending antenatal clinics are testing HIV-positive. For example, the sentinel surveillance data for the year 2002 show that several states, including Andhra Pradesh, Goa, Karnataka, Maharashtra, Manipur, Mizoram and Nagaland, have HIV prevalence rates of over 1 per cent among pregnant women (Bose, 2003). The increasing prevalence of HIV among pregnant women is likely to increase vertical transmission of the infection.

Endogenous and iatrogenic infections contribute significantly to the high prevalence of RTIs among women in India. For example, community-based studies among women in different parts of the country report a prevalence of bacterial vaginosis and candidiasis ranging from 14 per cent to 62 per cent and 1 per cent to 34 per cent respectively (Aggarwal et al., 1999; Bang et al., 1989; Bhatia et al., 1997; Garg et al., 2002; Mayank, Bahl and Bhandari, 2001; Nandan et al., 2001; Oomman, 1996; Prasad et al., 2000; Santhya, 1999).

Risk factors for RTI/STI/HIV transmission

Reliable data on the factors (proximate as well as background) placing men and women at risk of acquiring infection and the constraints they face in accessing appropriate and timely care are limited.

Factors related to sexual behaviour

Several factors related to sexual behaviour have led to a widespread and sustained epidemic of STIs, including HIV/AIDS in India. Sexual activity outside marriage is generally proscribed, but there has always been considerable laxity in favour of men. Several avenues, primarily commercial sex networks, are available for men seeking premarital and extramarital sexual relations. Cultural taboos on open discussion of sexual matters have constrained avenues for acquiring knowledge about safe sexual practices and the means for practising safe sex.

Sex workers

Several factors including high rates of partner change, early initiation into commercial sex, exposure to multiple STIs, non-use or limited use of condoms, and non-treatment or delayed or faulty treatment of STIs make sex workers a core group for the transmission of STIs, including HIV (Ramasubban, 2000).

A substantial proportion of female sex workers are young—one in three are below 25 years of age and almost one in ten are adolescents (NACO, 2001b). The vast majority are ever married, but often not currently living with their husbands. High partner change (three to five clients a day) characterises the sexual practices of sex workers (DFID et al, 2001a; Gangakhedkar et al., 1997; Ghosh and Das, 1990; Giri et al., 1995; Jacob, 1992; Jana, 1992; 1995; John et al., 1993). Studies show that men, particularly young men, often go to sex workers in groups and in such situations, the average number of penetrative episodes per sex worker may be even higher (Abraham, 1997; APAC, 1998b; Asthana and Oostvogels, 1996; Pelto, Joshi and Verma, 2000).

Given these high-risk practices, it is not surprising that the prevalence of STIs among sex workers is estimated to be high, ranging from 36 to 81 per cent (Venkataramana and Sarada, 2001). Studies show that HIV prevalence rates are also high; for example, 24 per cent in Goa and 55 per cent in Mumbai (Bose, 2003).

Clients of sex workers

Male clients of sex workers constitute a critical bridge population in spreading the infection from the core group to the general population. A substantial proportion of clients are below 25 years (two in five), ever married (more than one in two), and currently married and living with their spouse (two in five) (NACO, 2001b). By age 21, three-fourths had had their first sexual experience, with

7 per cent reporting sexual experience before 16 years. One in three reported sexual initiation with a sex worker. On an average, these men reported having sexual contact with 3.9 sex workers and 1.5 non-regular partners in the three months prior to the survey (NACO, 2001b). These sexual contacts, particularly those with non-regular partners, are often unprotected.

Mobile population groups such as truck crews are recognised as playing a major role in transmission (Bansal, 1992, 1995; George et al., 1997; Ramasubban, 2000; Singh and Malaviya, 1994; Singh et al., 1993; Solomon et al., 1998). A behavioural surveillance survey indicates that one-third of truck drivers and nearly one-half of helpers reported contact with sex workers in the year prior to the survey (DFID and FHI, 2001d). Small-scale studies report over 80 per cent of truckers visit sex workers regularly (two-seven times a week) and a substantial proportion engage in homosexual activities (Ahmed, 1992; Bryan, Fisher and Benziger, 2000; Rao et al., 1994, 1999; Singh and Malaviya, 1994). As may be expected, the prevalence of STIs among truckers is high, ranging from two-fifths to almost three-fourths (Gawande et al., 2000; Manjunath, Thappa and Jaisankar, 2002; Ramasubban, 2000).

Even though acknowledged as a potential bridge population, there has been little research on the social context or sexual behaviour of migrant groups in India (Ramasubban, 2000). Available evidence, however, reveals a serious lack of understanding of STI/HIV prevention and transmission (Gupta and Mitra, 1999), and high-risk practices including sexual contact with sex workers. More than one in ten clients of sex workers, for example, stay away from their regular residence (NACO, 2001b). These men run a high risk of spreading the infection to their sexual partners (Mukhopadhyay et al., 2001).

Drug users

Studies indicate that injecting drug users may constitute yet another bridge population due to drug use and unsafe sexual practices. Multiple partners are common and condom use is infrequent in this group (Chakrabarti et al., 2000; Eicher et al., 2000; Kumar et al., 2000a; NACO, 2002a; Panda et al., 1998; 2002; Sarkar et al., 1991; Sharma, Aggarwal and Dubey, 2002).

Men who have sex with men

Though not widely recognised, men who have sex with men (MSM) also constitute a bridge population for transmitting infection. Available evidence indicates that sexual contact among males is common in both rural and urban settings, and coercion is frequently reported (Pelto, 2000). Many men who engage in sex with men, including unmarried men, are involved in heterosexual activity as well (Khan, 1994; Kulkarni et al., 2000; NACO, 2002a; Pelto, 2000). Research indicates that almost one in three reported sex (often unprotected) with a female partner in the six months prior to the survey (NACO, 2002a). Sexual activity takes place in both commercial and non-commercial contexts (Chandiramani, 1998; Khan, 1994; Row Kavi, 1991).

Low-risk populations

Though premarital chastity and marital fidelity are still valued, a number of small-scale studies have observed comparatively high (at least, higher than culturally perceived) levels of premarital and extramarital sexual activity in the general population. A review of studies among young people reveals that fewer than 10 per cent of young women and 15-30 per cent of young men report premarital sexual experiences (Jejeebhoy and Sebastian, 2003). Sexual relations among young people tend to be characterised by early debut (particularly among women in the context of marriage), multiple partner and casual sexual relations, and visits to sex workers (particularly among young men), and lack of condom use (Jejeebhoy, 2002). Not surprisingly, between 7 and 22 per cent of male patients (the majority of whom were unmarried) and between

12 and 44 per cent of female patients (the majority of whom were married) attending STD clinics were reported to be adolescents (Chaudhary et al., 1988; Chopra et al., 1990; Siddappa, Kumar and Ravindra, 1990).

The extent of reported extramarital sexual activity (i.e., non-spousal sex reported by married people) is relatively low—2-6 per cent among women and 4-12 per cent among men (Basu, 1994; Collumbien et al., 2000; Kumar et al., 1997; Prasad et al., 2000; Santhya, 1999; Savara and Sridhar, 1994), although studies of STD clinic patients suggests that extramarital sexual activity may be higher in this group (Chaudhary et al., 1988; Chopra et al., 1990; Jacob et al., 1989; Kumar, Garg and Baruah, 1990; Siddappa, Kumar and Ravindra, 1990; Srikanth et al., 1997).

Limited use of condoms

Nationally, only 3.1 per cent of married couples were currently using condoms as a method of family planning in 1998-99 (IIPS and ORC Macro, 2000). Consistent use of condoms in non-marital sexual liaisons is also negligible among both high- and low-risk groups. Studies on premarital sexual behaviour among school- and college-age boys in India show that the vast majority are engaged in unprotected sex, even with commercial sex workers (Abraham and Kumar, 1999; Jejeebhoy, 2002; Selvan et al., 2001). In a study among sexually active unmarried and married men and women, but predominantly young, middle class, unmarried men in Mumbai, only 27 per cent reported always using condoms. Unmarried men and women are more likely to use condoms than their married counterparts (Roth, Krishnan and Bunch, 2001). Studies also show that condom use among young people is primarily motivated by the desire to prevent pregnancy rather than to prevent both STIs and pregnancy (Awasthi, Nichter and Pande, 2000; Collumbien, Das and Campbell, 2001). For example, in a study among unmarried and married men in Orissa, 19 per cent of sexually active unmarried men reported condom use during the last sexual act, and among those who reported condom use, 61 per cent reported pregnancy prevention as the main reason for use (Collumbien, Das and Campbell, 2001).

Studies among adults also show that 50-88 per cent of men who reported a non-marital sexual experience never used condoms during such encounters and a small proportion (4-13 per cent) reported that they always used condoms during non-marital sexual liaisons (Bloom et al., 2000; Collumbien et al., 2000; Kumar et al., 1997; Rajaram, 2000; Santhya, 1999).

Consistent condom use among perceived or known high-risk groups is also low. For example, a behavioural surveillance survey of sex workers indicates that only half reported consistent condom use with paying clients in the one month prior to the survey. The vast majority (80 per cent) of sex workers did not use condoms consistently with non-paying clients (NACO, 2001b).

Endogenous and iatrogenic factors

Studies documenting the role of endogenous and iatrogenic factors in causing RTIs are few in India. Evidence from these studies, though not definitely conclusive, indicates an association between the role of poor genital/personal hygiene and symptoms of RTIs (Bhatia and Cleland, 1995; Oomman, 1996; Santhya, 1999; Singh et al., 2001).

Among iatrogenic causes of infections, the use of IUDs has been reported to be a significant risk factor for pelvic inflammatory diseases in some facility-based studies (Shrikhande et al., 1995; Shrikhande, Zodpey and Kulkarni, 1998). Sterilised women are more likely to report experiencing lower or upper RTIs compared to non-users or users of reversible contraceptive methods (Bhatia and Cleland, 1995; Oomman, 1996). Studies also report that women who have undergone other invasive surgical procedures, including dilation and curettage, are more likely to experience pelvic inflammatory disease (Gogate et al., 1998).

Limited knowledge and misconceptions

While there is general awareness of HIV/AIDS, large sections of the population, particularly women and people in rural areas, are not aware of specific aspects such as the mode of transmission and the means of prevention. Nationally, for example, two in five rural women are not aware that HIV can be transmitted through sexual contact or blood transfusion. Similarly, fewer than one in two have complete knowledge of prevention, i.e., that consistent condom use and one faithful uninfected sexual partner are a means of preventing HIV/AIDS (NACO, 2001a). Evidence from small-scale studies reiterates these findings (Mawar et al., 1997; Singh, Bloom and Tsui, 1998).

Studies also show that incorrect knowledge and misconceptions are major barriers to consistent condom use (Balaiah et al., 1999; Sharma et al., 1997). Among truck drivers in Chennai, only 14 per cent know that using condoms could reduce HIV transmission, 13 per cent are aware that oil-based lubricants should not be used with condoms, and 59 per cent incorrectly believe that condoms only need to be used with sex workers; however, 92 per cent know it is unsafe to reuse a condom (Bryan, Fisher and Benziger, 2000).

Perceptions/misperceptions often rooted in cultural and ethno-medical beliefs may also place men and women at risk of engaging in high-risk behaviours or not adopting protective behaviours. Explorations of young men's sexual anxieties and health problems in Gujarat indicate that most perceive semen loss through masturbation and nocturnal emissions as dangerous, leading to weakness and impotence. Some young men feel that they must seek out sexual partners, including sex workers, to avoid the debilitating effects of semen loss (Deepak Charitable Trust, 2000).

Gender inequalities and norms

Gender inequalities and women's relative lack of autonomy in matters relating to their lives influence their risk of acquiring infections in several ways (Bharat and Aggleton, 1999; Jejeebhoy and Koenig, 2003; Mane and Maitra, 1992; Ramasubban, 2000). Women who are socially, culturally and economically dependent and subordinate to their sexual partners may find it difficult to make decisions on whether or not to have sex, or to negotiate and convince partners to have safe sex within and outside of marriage (George and Jaswal, 1995; Santhya and Dasvarma, 2002). A community-based study reports that two-thirds of symptomatic women who requested their husbands not to have sex were either verbally abused or beaten (Santhya and Dasvarma, 2002). Sex workers are also constrained from exercising their sexual and reproductive rights (Ramasubban, 2000).

Lack of intimacy or partner communication which makes talking about sex, pregnancy and safe practices extremely difficult may also make sexual partners particularly female partners vulnerable to infections (Jejeebhoy and Koenig, 2003). Several studies show that women and men often do not inform their spouses about their gynaecological symptoms (Bang and Bang, 1994; Marfatia et al., 2000; Ramasubban and Rishyasringa, 2000; Sahasrabuddhe et al., 2002; Santhya and Dasvarma, 2002). A study among married women and men in rural Tamil Nadu reported that slightly more than one-third (37.3 per cent) of women with symptoms of possible RTIs and one-fifth (19.9 per cent) of symptomatic men informed their spouses about their illness experience (Santhya and Dasvarma, 2002).

Prevailing norms of masculinity and femininity may reinforce risk behaviours (Jejeebhoy and Koenig, 2003). Dominant ideologies of masculinity may prevent boys and men from seeking information on sex for fear of appearing ignorant and therefore unmanly, and at the same time, may condone gaining sexual experience through liaisons with girlfriends and sex workers. In contrast, dominant ideologies of femininity may silence the voices of women, who could be fearful that their reputation is at stake if they appear too knowledgeable about sexual matters or play an active role in sexual relationships.

Health care seeking behaviour

While currently available studies of men and women with RTIs/STIs or symptoms suggestive of these infections have shed light on their patterns of health care seeking, the constraints that they face in accessing appropriate and timely care are less well understood (Hawkes and Santhya, 2001).

Pattern of treatment-seeking

There are wide variations in patterns of treatment-seeking for RTIs/STIs. However, a common observation is that a significant proportion of symptomatic men and women do not seek treatment. Studies report that between one-third and two-third of women suffering from symptoms suggestive of RTIs/STIs do not seek treatment (Barua, 2000; Bhatia and Cleland, 2001; IIPS and ORC Macro, 2000; Oomman, 1996; Prasad et al., 2000; Ravindran, 1995b; Sadhu et al., 2001; Santhya, 1999). When care is sought, it tends to be after some delay (Ramasubban and Rishyasringa, 2000; Santhya, 1999).

Women often seek medical intervention only when they find they are too weak to work or experience problems in their sexual relationships (APAC, 1998b; Kotecha et al., 1999). Even when treatment is sought, women tend to follow a sequence of options, ranging from self-treatment or home remedies to visiting traditional healers, unqualified practitioners or qualified allopathic providers (Jejeebhoy and Koenig, 2003; Oomman, 2000; Ramasubban, 2000). Non-compliance with the recommended treatment regimen is not uncommon (Singh et al., 2001). Adolescent girls tend to be even more reluctant to seek treatment for symptoms suggestive of RTIs/STIs (Andrew and Patel, 2002; Barua and Kurz, 2001; Prasad et al., 2000; Santhya and Jejeebhoy, 2003).

Less is known about the health-seeking behaviour of men in the general population. Studies report that men also suffer in silence or resort to self-treatment for STIs (Santhya, 1999; Verma et al., 2000). A few studies, however, report that between one-half and all symptomatic men consult someone or seek allopathic treatment (Carolina Population Centre, 1997; Joseph et al., 1998). Non-compliance with the treatment regimen and self-treatment are common among men as well (Ganguli et al., 1985). It is reported that over one-half of cases seen at larger public hospitals are repeat patients who come with persistent or aggravated symptoms after considerable 'cure-shopping' (Ramasubban, 2000).

Data on treatment-seeking patterns among high-risk population groups indicate that inaction is not as widespread among these groups as compared to the general population. However, self-treatment with home remedies, over-the-counter drugs, treatment from traditional healers or unqualified practitioners, resort to multiple sources of treatment and non-compliance with the recommended treatment regimen are common (APAC, 1998b; 2001; Evans and Lambert, 1997; NACO, 2001b; 2002a).

Quality of services

While several contextual and individual level factors contribute to poor health care seeking practices, health system level factors including the lack of quality services, inadequate accessibility and high cost also play a significant role.

The quality, availability and access to health care for RTIs/STIs remain a critical research area that has not been adequately explored. Available evidence reveals that the quality of RTI/STI care continues to be poor. Recommended case management guidelines are not often followed in diagnosis (APAC, 1999; DFID et al., 2001g; 2001h; 2001i; 2001j; 2001k; Mertens et al., 1998). Similarly, in most cases, providers do not follow prescribed treatment regimens. Recommended co-treatment to cover common causes of STI symptoms is rarely given. In a study of male patients with genital ulcers in Chennai, for example, only 12 per cent received effective treatment against both syphilis and chancroid (Kantharaj et al., 1995). Moreover, where effective antibiotics are prescribed, both over-treatment and under-treatment are common, with most providers prescribing excessive doses (DFID et al., 2001g).

The quality of counselling for STI prevention is inadequate in STD clinics in both the public and private sector (DFID et al., 2001g; 2001h; 2001i; 2001j; DFID and FHI, 2001e; Marfatia et al., 2000; Mertens et al., 1998; Nataraj, 1994; Roy et al., 1998). A multi-state study shows that fewer than one in five providers advised patients on condom use. Compared to public sector providers, a higher proportion of private practitioners provided advice on condom use (DFID et al., 2001g; 2001h; 2001i; 2001j; DFID and FHI, 2001e). Observations of STI consultations in Chennai revealed that instructions on how to use condoms were given to 6 per cent of clients, and condoms provided to only 1 per cent (Mertens et al., 1998).

Although partner notification is the cornerstone of effective STI management, this issue is rarely discussed or initiated by health care providers (DFID et al., 2001g; 2001h; 2001i; 2001j; DFID and FHI, 2001e; Mertens et al., 1998; Roy et al., 1998; Santhya and Dasvarma, 2002). A clinic-based study in Chennai shows that advice on partner notification was given during only 27 per cent of the consultations (Mertens et al., 1998). In a community-based study in rural Tamil Nadu, none of the symptomatic (suggestive of RTIs) women and only 5.7 per cent of the symptomatic men were advised to have their spouses examined for a possible infection (Santhya and Dasvarma, 2002).

An overwhelming majority of men and women with RTIs/STIs seek care from informal providers for reasons of secrecy, absence of physical examination or follow-up (Ramasubban, 2000). The quality of services provided by these informal providers is inadequate and does not differ substantially from that of formal providers (APAC, 1999; DFID et al., 2001g; 2001h; 2001i; 2001j).

Apart from the poor technical quality of services, studies also show that the intimidating and judgmental attitudes of providers prevent many from seeking care from formal providers (Santhya and Dasvarma, 2002).

Access to services

Access to RTI/STI services is grossly inadequate, particularly in rural areas. With the shift in the reproductive health paradigm, there have been efforts to integrate services for the treatment of RTIs/STIs at all levels of health care, including at the primary health care level. However, primary health care facilities are currently inadequately equipped to offer effective diagnosis and treatment for RTIs/STIs. For example, a recent survey of health facilities across the country reports that RTI/STI services are provided by only one-sixth of primary health centres as most lack trained staff and facilities. Only 46 per cent of these centres have a laboratory and in several states, fewer than one-fifth have a laboratory. The survey also indicates that there is a mismatch between the availability of laboratory facilities and laboratory technicians—for example, in Maharashtra, while 97 per cent of the primary health centres have laboratories, only 24 per cent have a laboratory technician on the staff. In West Bengal, in contrast, while only 4 per cent of primary health centres have a laboratory, 20 per cent have a laboratory technician. Additionally, only 25 per cent of primary health centres have at least one medical officer trained in RTI/STI treatment. Moreover, most primary health centres (82 per cent) do not have a female medical officer (IIPS, 2001b), which may severely constrain women's ability to access RTI/STI services, even if made available at the primary health centre level. Facilities for the diagnosis and treatment of RTIs/STIs are far from adequate even at the level of community health centres, first referral units and districts hospital that are expected to function as referral units (IIPS, 2001b).

Cost of services

The high cost of seeking care for RTIs/STIs could be a major obstacle for many men and women. However, evidence on the cost of RTI/STI services is sparse in India. A recent survey of household level expenditure on reproductive and child health care in Rajasthan shows that families spend more of their own money on seeking care for symptoms of RTIs than they spend on child health care and services for safe motherhood (pre- and post-natal, obstetric, and abortion) (IIHMR, 2000). A study in Karnataka reports that treatment of genito-urinary problems accounted for one-fourth of annual expenditure and these together with problems related to pregnancy or family planning accounted for one-third (Bhatia and Cleland, 2001).

Programme response

With the emergence of the HIV epidemic, programme efforts to control the spread of RTIs/STIs have been significantly enhanced. Major programmatic responses are discussed briefly in the following sections.

Surveillance activities

In response to the emergence of HIV epidemic, there have been some efforts to improve the surveillance activities in the country. Several centres for HIV surveillance have been established. Currently, there are 384 sentinel sites—165 sites in STD clinics, 200 sites in antenatal clinics, 14 sites for injecting drug users, 3 sites for MSM and 2 sites for sex workers (Joshi, 2003). STI surveillance through syndrome-based information from the primary health centres and aetiological information from STD clinics is planned, though not yet started. Behavioural surveillance has been incorporated into national HIV surveillance activities recently and the first round of surveys was conducted in 2001-02. State-level behavioural surveillance surveys have also been conducted in selected states including Tamil Nadu (where the first wave of behavioural surveillance surveys in India was initiated in 1996), Andhra Pradesh, Gujarat, Kerala, Maharashtra, Orissa and West Bengal.

STI case management

Several measures were adopted in the 1990s to strengthen the STI control programme, most significantly the effort to integrate STI services into the existing health care system, particularly at the primary health centre level. Simplified STI Treatment Guidelines were developed and health care providers at the primary care levels trained in syndromic management of STIs to facilitate this integration (NACO, 1998). NACO has recently updated the guidelines for diagnosis and case management (NACO, 2003b). However, the effectiveness of syndromic management of STIs in women is currently being questioned. Studies indicate that the use of recommended syndromic flow charts may lead to the poor management of STIs in both low- and high-risk population groups in India (DFID et al, 2001a; 2001b; 2001c; 2001d; 2001e; 2001f; Vishwanath et al., 2000).

Other public health interventions for STI control, such as screening pregnant women for syphilis and ophthalmia neonatorum, are implemented erratically throughout the country (Hawkes and Santhya, 2001).

STI prevention and care outside the public sector

NGOs have often taken the lead in promoting behaviour change communication and safe sex initiatives, providing counselling and treatment for STIs and home-based care for people living with HIV/AIDS. A leading example of STI/HIV prevention and management through behaviour change communication is the Sonagachi intervention among sex workers in Kolkata (DMSC, 1998). Recognising the importance of forging partnerships with NGOs and community-based organisations (CBOs), NACO has supported several NGOs, formulated guidelines for an open and transparent system of selection of NGOs, and decentralised funding of NGOs to State AIDS Control Societies.

Voluntary HIV counselling and testing

The Government of India's policy statement on HIV testing emphasises that no individual should undergo mandatory testing for HIV, adequate voluntary testing facilities with pre- and post-test counselling should be made available throughout the country, there should be at least one government-run HIV testing centre per district, and results should be kept strictly confidential, apart from the spouse or sexual partner of the person undergoing the test (NACO, 2002b). Currently, however, most persons undergoing HIV testing are referred rather than voluntary. The focus of counselling is on prevention and awareness generation rather than on a continuum between prevention and care and support. Counselling is individual-centred rather family-oriented. Above all, the very name of voluntary testing and counselling evokes stigma (Ghosh, 2003).

Care and support for people living with HIV/AIDS

The government, NGOs and international organisations like WHO have taken several measures to provide quality care and support to people living with HIV/AIDS. For example, NACO, in collaboration with WHO and local NGOs, has been conducting pilot programmes on care and support for people living with HIV/AIDS in Maharashtra, Manipur and Tamil Nadu. The NGO sector has established model care and support programmes for people living with HIV/AIDS in many of the larger cities (Population Council, 2002).

Despite these measures, studies show that hospitals and other care settings are the main sites where HIV-positive people face discrimination and stigma (Bharat, 1999). Compounding these problems is the exorbitant cost of most treatment options. A cohort study of HIV/AIDS clients on anti-retroviral (ARV) and non-ARV treatment in Chennai shows that the average financial burden of treatment, measured as a percentage of monthly household income spent on treatment and services, is 49 per cent, which in the case of low-income households is as high as 82 per cent (Duraisamy et al., 2003). Currently no subsidies for the purchase of antiretroviral drugs are available, though the government has been progressively reducing the excise and customs duties on these drugs.

The way forward

Although it is difficult to precisely estimate the prevalence of RTIs/STIs in India, evidence suggests that a large number of people are getting infected annually. Efforts to gather evidence on the magnitude and pattern of RTIs/STIs and related risk factors have increased significantly over the past decade. However, several gaps in our understanding continue to constrain the design of appropriate responses to contain these infections. While policy and programmatic responses for the prevention and control of these infections have expanded, these remain focused narrowly on selected population groups, their implementation patchy, and their effectiveness inadequately documented or evaluated. Critical issues to be addressed to improve the evidence-base and design appropriate responses for the prevention and control of RTIs/STIs in the country are highlighted.

Programme recommendations

- The current systems for surveillance of STIs/HIV, although expanded, do not provide a complete picture of the incidence/prevalence of these infections or trends over time. Surveillance activities in rural areas need to be expanded and mechanisms devised to gather data from private sector providers.
- Although targeted interventions have been successful in certain geographical areas, Sonagachi for example, and among selected high-risk groups, their coverage remains limited. Several not-so-easily reachable population groups, such as non-brothel-based sex workers and migrants, continue to remain outside the focus of interventions. Similarly, although young people are increasingly engaging in high-risk practices, programmes directed at young people are limited. It is crucial that interventions are designed to cover hitherto under-served population groups. Equally important is to adopt a continuum approach that goes beyond prevention and control to care and support.

- Policy prescriptions for integrating RTI/STI management with basic health services at the primary health care level have been clearly outlined. However, the capacity of the primary health care system remains limited. Hence, there is a need to strengthen the basic infrastructure, ensure the availability of trained manpower at different levels of health care as well as delivery of high quality and humane services.

Research recommendations

- Our understanding of the prevalence of RTIs/STIs and factors placing men and women at risk of these infections continues to be primarily limited to selected high-risk groups. Many high-risk, but not-so-easily approachable groups such as non-brothel-based sex workers, sex workers in rural areas and small towns, men who have sex with men, drug users and mobile/migrant population groups have not been adequately studied. Focused data are needed to understand the STI situation and behaviours of these groups so that appropriate responses for the prevention and control of STIs/HIV among them could be designed.
- Estimating the incidence/prevalence of RTIs/STIs and accurately using available data is extremely difficult given the highly divergent nature of studies and laboratory methods used. The need for standardisation of laboratory methods is particularly crucial for any future studies.
- Despite extensive promotional campaigns, condom use continues to be negligible within and outside marriage, and the acceptability of the condom as a dual protection method remains low. Social science research to understand people's perceptions of dual protection needs and the strategies that men and women adopt to meet these needs and operational research to test ways to effectively promote condoms as a dual protection method among all population groups, especially among young people, are critical. Similarly, with new prophylactic methods being developed, studies on user perspectives

will provide valuable insights for introducing these methods in the country.

- The role of endogenous factors in contributing to the high prevalence of RTIs remains relatively unexplored. Emerging evidence that endogenous infections such as bacterial vaginosis may facilitate HIV transmission highlights the need for research on the prevalence of these infections in low- and high-risk population groups. The role of over-use of antibiotics, poor nutritional status and other endogenous factors also need to be explored. Similarly, further research is required on the association between invasive trans-cervical procedures and the transmission of RTIs as current evidence is limited and inconclusive.
- Research is needed that highlights the pathways through which prevailing norms predispose men and women to engage in high-risk practices or adopt protective behaviours. Similarly, studies exploring the ways in which gender inequalities increase women's vulnerability are needed to design holistic programmes for improving women's reproductive health.
- While currently available studies shed some light on the patterns of health care seeking for RTI/STI symptoms, the socio-cultural and system-level constraints that men and women face in acquiring services (and, hence, opportunities to intervene) are less well understood. The role of a wide variety of possible influences (monetary, geographical, gender-based personal relations, perceptions on the quality of care, etc) has yet to be appreciated.
- Although the current syndromic management of RTIs/STIs is justified, it is important to assess the clinical, cost and operational effectiveness of this strategy so that necessary modifications can be effected. Equally important is to test the feasibility and effectiveness of other strategies including presumptive treatment in high-risk population groups.

Young People's Sexual and Reproductive Health

Shireen J. Jejeebhoy and Mary Philip Sebastian

There are an estimated 300 million young people (aged 10-24 years) in India today comprising almost one-third (31 per cent) of the country's population. Specifically, 22 per cent of India's population falls into the adolescent age group (aged 10-19) (IIPS and ORC Macro, 2000; United Nations, 2001).

Young people are healthier, more urbanised and better educated than earlier generations; they experience puberty at younger ages, and marry and have children later than in the past. At the same time, they face significant risks related to sexual and reproductive health, and many lack the power to make informed sexual and reproductive choices. These vulnerabilities remain poorly understood.

The context of sexual relations among young people

Young people in India are a heterogeneous group and their situation varies widely by age, gender, marital status, class, region,

---

This chaptere is an abriged version of a working paper by Shireen J.Jejeebhoy and Mary Philip Sebastian titled 'Actions that Protect: Promotong Sexual and Reproductive Health and Choice among Young People in India' (2003).

state and cultural context. These variations call for interventions that are flexible and responsive to their disparate needs. A socio-demographic profile of young people in India suggests that a significant proportion remain illiterate. Wide geographic and gender disparities in enrolment are reflected: for example, among adolescents aged 15-17, 63 per cent of those living in urban areas attend school, compared to 44 per cent in rural areas. School attendance varies widely by state—while over 90 per cent of those aged 6-17 were in school in Himachal Pradesh and Kerala, only 60 per cent were in school in Bihar (IIPS and ORC Macro, 2000). Gender disparities are also stark. While 15 per cent of young males aged 15-19 are illiterate, about twice this percentage (32 per cent) of females are illiterate. And while 58 per cent of young males in the eligible ages are enrolled in middle and secondary school, only 40 per cent of young females are (IIPS and ORC Macro, 2000). Even so, the proportion of women aged 20-24 who report seven or more years of education (34 per cent) is dramatically higher than the proportion of older women aged 40-44 who do so (18 per cent) (Singh, 1998).

A substantial proportion of young people are economically active. By ages 15-19, large proportions of young boys (44 per cent) and girls (26 per cent) are engaged in economic activity; however these figures may not adequately reflect girls' contributions to household labour. Rural adolescents are more likely to work and less likely to study than their urban counterparts (ILO, 1998).

Mortality rates among young people are generally lower than those observed at younger and older ages, a reflection of the fact that youth is a generally healthy period of life. However, gender disparities are apparent, particularly among young people aged 15-19 (2.5 and 1.8, respectively per 1,000 females and males) and 20-24 (3.8 and 2.7 per 1,000 respectively), and may be explained by the poorer reproductive health of young women at these ages (IIPS and ORC Macro, 2000).

Sexual relations among young people tend to be characterised by early debut (particularly among women in the context of marriage), multiple partners and casual sexual relations (particularly among young males), lack of contraception or condom use, and coercion and non-consensual experiences.

Table 7

Percentage of young women married by age 13, 15, 18 years

	Women currently aged:	
	20-24	*25-29*
Proportion ever married	78.8	94.5
Percentage married by age 13	8.9	12.1
Percentage married by age 15	23.5	29.2
Percentage married by age 18	50.0	58.9
Percentage married in adolescence (by age 20)	67.1	74.9

Source: IIPS and ORC Macro, 2000.

Onset of sexual relations within marriage

While international attention tends to focus on *premarital* sexual activity among young people, for young women in India, sexual relations occur overwhelmingly within the context of marriage (see Pelto, Joshi and Verma, 2000). Despite rising age at marriage and laws prohibiting early marriage, half of all women aged 20-24 are married by 18 years, and a quarter by 15 years (see Table 7) (IIPS and ORC Macro, 2000; Santhya and Jejeebhoy, 2003). In contrast, boys rarely marry as adolescents (only 6 per cent of adolescent boys were married) (IIPS and ORC Macro, 2000; Kulkarni, 2003).

There is considerable state-wise variation in age at marriage (IIPS and ORC Macro, 2000). Early marriage is concentrated in the large northern states of Bihar (and Jharkhand), Madhya Pradesh (and Chhatisgarh), Rajasthan and Uttar Pradesh (and Uttaranchal). In these states, and in Andhra Pradesh in the south, over 40 per cent of all girls aged 15-19 are already married; moreover, 40 per cent or more women aged 20-24 were already married by age 15. While marriage among males takes place far more rarely in adolescence, it is these same states in which between 10 per cent and 21 per cent of those aged 15-19 are already married.

Premarital sexual relations

While marriage marks the onset of sexual activity among the large majority of young women, there is growing evidence of premarital onset of sexual activity particularly among young men. Evidence from small studies, which may be unrepresentative of the general population, suggests that 0-10 per cent of young women and 15-30 per cent of young men reported premarital sexual experience (see Figure 4) (Abraham and Kumar, 1999; Awasthi, Nichter and Pande, 2000; Jejeebhoy, 2000a). There may, however, be some over-reporting among males and some underreporting among females. Among young men and women who are sexually active, age at sexual debut occurs in late adolescence.

Figure 4

Premarital sexual activity among youth: Selected studies, 1990s

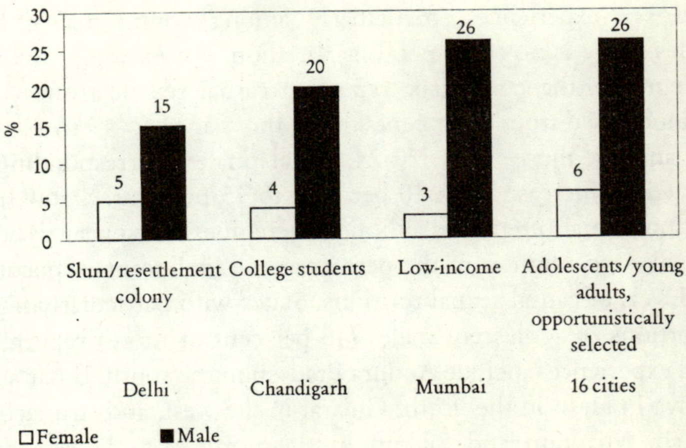

Source: Abraham and Kumar 1999 for Mumbai; Kaur et al., 1996 for Chandigarh; Mehra, Savithri and Coutinho 2002 for Delhi; Watsa 1993 for the 16 city study.

Sexual relations: How risky?

Casual and sex worker relations

The nature of premarital partnerships differs markedly between young men and women. The majority of sexually experienced unmarried women reported having sex with a steady partner with marriage in mind (see Brown et al., 2001). In contrast, a significant proportion of young men who tend to report sexual debut at ages 16-19 reported multiple partners, casual partners, visits to commercial sex workers and 'aunties'—older married women in the neighbourhood (Abraham and Kumar, 1999; Goparaju, 1993; Jejeebhoy, 2000a; Savara and Sridhar, 1993; Sharma and Sharma, 1996; Sodhi and Verma, forthcoming).

Variations by region, age and state are reflected in casual sex relations. According to the recent NACO National Behavioural Surveillance Survey, some 10 per cent and 8 per cent of rural and urban young men aged 15-19, respectively, reported a casual sex encounter in the 12 months preceding the survey compared to 2 per cent of sexually active young rural and urban females (NACO and UNICEF, 2002). Age appears to be associated with increased casual sex experiences, particularly among young males; for females, there is no corresponding variation. For example, among urban males, the percentage reporting casual sex in a one-year recall increased from 8 per cent among those aged 15-19 to 13 per cent among those aged 20-24; rural males correspondingly reported an increase from 10 per cent to 15 per cent. State-wise variations are also reported although there does not appear to be a regional concentration in the percentage of adolescents reporting high levels of causal sexual relations. States with particularly high proportions of adolescent males (15 per cent or more) reporting casual experiences include Andhra Pradesh in the south, Bihar and Madhya Pradesh in the north, Gujarat in the west, and Arunachal Pradesh, Mizoram and Sikkim in the north-east. Those with particularly high proportions of young females (5 per cent or more) reporting a casual experience include Andhra Pradesh and Kerala in the south, Bihar in the north, Maharashtra in the west, and Arunachal Pradesh and Nagaland in the north-east.

Lack of contraceptive or condom use

Lack of contraceptive or condom use and discontinuation and failure rates characterise the vast majority of sexual encounters among youth, and consequently rates of unplanned pregnancy are high (Singh, 1998). For example, only 8 per cent of married women aged 15-19 were using any method of contraception at the time of the NFHS 2 survey and 5 per cent were using a modern method. Regional variation in contraceptive practice is relatively narrow in these ages—notable are such states as Punjab and West Bengal in which 17 per cent and 33 per cent of currently married adolescents respectively reported current contraceptive practice. As a result, some 15 per cent of births among adolescents aged 15-19 were reportedly unplanned (Pachauri and Santhya, 2003). Indeed, 27 per cent expressed an unmet need for contraception (IIPS and ORC Macro, 2000). Considerable state-wise variation is observed as a result of differential family size preferences and access to contraceptive supplies: unmet need is reported by under 10 per cent of adolescents in Punjab and Haryana and by around one-third or more in such states as Bihar, Jammu and Kashmir, Rajasthan, Maharashtra and even Kerala (IIPS and ORC Macro, 2000).

Few studies have explored contraceptive or condom use by the unmarried, and those that do report largely on young males. Contraceptive use is generally infrequent and irregular. Only one in three (32 per cent) of sexually experienced adolescent men in a slum setting in Lucknow reported condom use in relations with sex workers and approximately half (56 per cent) in relations with a friend or relative (Awasthi, Nichter and Pande, 2000). Among truck cleaners in Indore, almost all (93 per cent) of the sexually active had never used condoms in their relations with sex workers (Bansal, 1992). College students were more likely to report condom use, although less than half the sexually active had ever used a condom or any other form of contraception, and even fewer did so regularly or with all partners (Abraham and Kumar, 1999). They were also more likely to report contraceptive/condom use in contacts with sex workers than in relations with regular or 'casual' partners. However, they rarely reported regular use of any method (Abraham and Kumar, 1999; Joseph, Prasad and Abraham, 2003). The main reasons for the non-use of condoms were the spontaneity of sex, lack of awareness of the condom and how to procure it, and the perception that condom use reduces pleasure.

Lack of consistent condom use within casual relationships among youth has been reported at the national level (NACO and UNICEF, 2002). About half of young females and males reporting casual sex reported using a condom at the last sexual encounter; however, only 25 per cent and 37 per cent of males and 24 per cent and 28 per cent of females aged 15-19 in rural and urban areas, respectively, reported consistent condom use in all casual encounters in the 12 months preceding the survey. State-wise variation is evident but by and large, fewer than half of all those reporting a casual sexual experience report consistent condom use in most states.

Non-consensual sexual activity among adolescents

Although rarely reported, evidence suggests that a number of adolescent girls and boys are subjected to forced sexual relations. A study of school-going adolescents in Goa found that 7 per cent of boys and 6 per cent of girls reported forced sexual relations and one-third reported some kind of unwanted touch (Patel and Andrew, 2001). For a substantial minority of women, sexual initiation was accompanied by force and fear, both in and out of marriage. However, experiences may be underreported (Sodhi and Verma, 2003).

Married women also experience coercion. Early sexual encounters with their husbands may be traumatic and forced reflecting the vulnerability of the newly married (George and Jaswal, 1995; Khan et al., 1997). The exercise of sexual choice is

Non-consensual sexual relations are reported by married females

"I decided to stop it since I used to feel uneasy while having sex with a big abdomen. But my husband used to get angry if I told him that I did not want to have sex. He used to tell me that he would remarry if I refused to have sex with him. I tried to explain to him, but he did not want to listen….

"I had to give in to his demands after a few days and our tiffs were resolved. We continued in this manner till my ninth month. I had feelings of discomfort but I had to accept my husband's wishes."

Source: 18-year-old woman who had recently delivered a child (Santhya, McGrory and Haberland, 2001).

sometimes met with marital conflict and threats of remarriage (Santhya, McGrory and Haberland, 2001).

Young men and boys also experience non-consensual sex. While young men are often reluctant to admit the experience of forced sex, studies indicate that 6-7 per cent of boys and young men reported a coercive experience, usually perpetrated by an older male (Patel and Andrew, 2001). Street boys in Bangalore reported that they were initiated into coerced sex at an early age, usually perpetrated by an older male (Ramakrishna, Karott and Murthy, 2003).

Associated risk behaviours

Studies in India, while relatively sparse, have recognised the links between substance abuse injuries and violence and impaired capacity to make decisions on safe sexual behaviour. For example, in a study of adolescent boys in urban slums in Lucknow, substance abuse was reported by a substantial minority, and was associated with irregular condom use and STI (Awasthi and Pande, 1998). Likewise, a study of adolescent truck cleaners reported that of 210 adolescent boys interviewed, cigarettes were commonly used, and a minority reported extensive use of chewing tobacco, opium and alcohol; links with unprotected sexual relations were also observed (Bansal, 1992). The study of sexual coercion among school-going adolescents in Goa referred to above also reports a significant association between substance abuse and sexual coercion (Patel and Andrew, 2001).

Reproductive health outcomes

Pregnancy and childbearing

Pregnancy and childbearing characterise the experiences of a number of young women in India. Adolescent fertility rates are high: roughly 107 births take place per 1,000 girls aged 15-19 and the fertility of this age group makes up 19 per cent of the nation's total fertility rate (IIPS and ORC Macro, 2000). Over one in five give birth by age 17 and the median age at first birth is 19 years, suggesting that significant proportions of women undergo pregnancy at ages below which obstetric risks are particularly elevated. Not only does childbearing occur early among married adolescents, but subsequent pregnancies also tend to be more closely spaced than among adults (Santhya and Jejeebhoy, 2003). The experience of early and closely spaced childbearing is particularly risky for adolescents because large proportions are anaemic and may not have reached physical maturity—nearly 15 per cent of ever-married adolescent women are stunted, and about one-fifth have moderate to severe anaemia (IIPS and ORC Macro, 2000).

Early childbearing has resulted in adverse health consequences, including damage to the reproductive tract, maternal mortality, pregnancy complications, peri-natal and neonatal mortality and low birth weight (Kulkarni, 2003). Evidence from community- and facility-based studies reiterate that maternal deaths are considerably higher among adolescents than older women. Estimates derived from a community-based study in rural Andhra Pradesh indicate that in the 1980s the maternal mortality ratio experienced by adolescents was almost twice that of women aged 25-39 years (Bhatia, 1993). Hospital-based studies reiterate these differences. A national study conducted by Indian Council of Medical Research of 43,550 women in 10 facilities reports that maternal mortality among adolescents was 645 per 100,000 live births, compared to 342 per 100,000 births in adult women aged 20-34 years (Krishna, 1995). Similarly, a study in Mumbai indicates that while the maternal mortality ratio among women aged 20-29 was 138 per 100,000 live births, adolescents experienced considerably higher ratios—206 per 100,000 live births (Pachauri and Jamshedji, 1983). Neonatal mortality, a key outcome of unsafe pregnancy conditions, is significantly higher among adolescent mothers than among those aged 20-29: 63.1 and 21.2 per 1,000 live births, respectively (IIPS and ORC Macro, 2000).

NFHS 2 data indicate disparities between the large northern and eastern states and the rest of India with regard to neonatal mortality: such states as Bihar, Madhya Pradesh, Orissa, Rajasthan and Uttar Pradesh continue to experience exceptionally high rates of neonatal mortality among adolescent (and older) mothers. State-wise variation is less marked in the case of other key indicators such as median age at first pregnancy and extent of anaemia among married adolecents, although it is Kerala that reveals the highest median age at first pregnancy and lowest proportions of anaemic adolescents.

Induced abortion

As abortion is such a sensitive topic, levels of induced abortion are difficult to measure directly. However, small studies suggest that a substantial proportion of adolescents, both married and unmarried, seek abortion services. It is estimated that between 1 and 10 per cent of abortion-seekers in India are adolescents (Ganatra, 2000), though a few facility-based studies report that the proportion of adolescent abortion-seekers is as high as one in three (Chhabra et al., 1988; Solapurkar and Sangam, 1985). An analysis of data from NFHS 1998-99 shows a lifetime induced abortion ratio of 1.1 among married adolescents nationally (Pachauri and Santhya, 2002b). Among unmarried abortion-seekers, adolescents constitute a disproportionately large percentage of those who seek abortions. At least one-half of unmarried women seeking abortions are adolescents, many of whom are below 15 years (Jejeebhoy, 2000a). A community-based study in rural Maharashtra reports that young women aged 15-24 constituted over half of married abortion-seekers in the area (Ganatra and Hirve, 2002b). Findings of this study suggest, moreover, that adolescents have considerably less decision-making authority than older abortion-seekers, are more likely to be coerced into an abortion, or conversely, to face opposition from their families, and are more likely to report post-abortion morbidity.

Reproductive tract and sexually transmitted infections

Few studies have specifically addressed RTIs or STIs among young people. The National Behavioural Surveillance Survey of the National AIDS Control Organisation indicates that approximately 3 per cent of young males and 5 per cent of young females reported the experience of symptoms of infection (STIs or RTIs more generally) such as discharge, ulcers or sores in the 12 months preceding the survey. These figures undoubtedly reflect considerable under-reporting (NACO and UNICEF, 2002). A community-based study of RTI prevalence among married women aged 16-22 in rural Tamil Nadu underscores the extent to which infections go unnoticed in this outwardly 'low-risk' population. Forty-nine per cent of women in the study reported experiencing symptoms of RTIs, while clinical and laboratory examination diagnosed 18 per cent with an STI (Joseph, Prasad and Abraham, 2003).

A significant finding is that husbands' behaviour may transmit infection to their wives, which could have serious implications given that many infected women are asymptomatic and are unlikely to seek care even when symptoms appear (Joseph, Prasad and Abraham, 2003).

In several settings HIV rates among 15-24-year-olds are equal to or in excess of those estimated among adults. In India, for example, rates for young women exceed those for both young men and adults (0.96 per cent, 0.46 per cent and 0.80 per cent respectively) (UNICEF, UNAIDS and WHO, 2002).

Underlying risk and protective factors

A host of factors may inhibit young people from achieving good sexual and reproductive health. Many are structural, such as poverty and malnutrition, patriarchy, early marriage and inadequate educational and health systems, and, in turn, influence risk and protective factors at the individual level. The range of obstacles observed to prevent young people from achieving good health and exercising informed choices are outlined below.

Limited awareness of health promoting behaviours

While awareness of contraception and infection may be almost universal at a superficial level, in-depth awareness of sexual health issues, health promoting actions and risky sexual behaviour is limited among young people. A study reports for example, that although a large proportion of adolescent girls and boys had heard of STIs (66 per cent and 87 per cent, respectively) and contraception (91 per cent and 94 per cent, respectively), only 2 per cent could name an STI apart from HIV/AIDS, and only 37 per cent of girls, compared to 84 per cent of boys, were aware that condoms can provide protection against infection (Sebastian et al., 2002a).

The NACO National Behavioural Surveillance Survey discloses that although 90 per cent of young men and 80 per cent of young women aged 15-19 had heard of HIV/AIDS, state-wise variations are considerable, particularly among females. For example, fewer than 40 per cent of rural women (particularly those aged 15-19) in such states as Bihar, Gujarat, Jharkhand, Madhya Pradesh and Uttar Pradesh were aware of HIV. This awareness did not translate into in-depth knowledge of symptoms, modes of transmission or methods of prevention. In general, only 60 and 54 per cent of urban and rural males aged 15-19 and 56 and 45 per cent of females could accurately identify two modes of prevention, and only 58 per cent of young women and men were aware that there is no cure. Awareness of STIs and their links to HIV was even more limited: 28 per cent of young men and 29 per cent of young women had heard of STIs, and only 21 per cent and 18 per cent respectively were aware that STI patients have a higher risk of HIV infection than others. Again, state-wise variations are evident. Significant disparities are also observed by education and marital status. As expected, better-educated youth are consistently more aware of HIV and protective factors than are others. The unmarried are more likely to be aware of HIV than the married, suggesting that married women may be particularly poorly aware and vulnerable (NACO and UNICEF, 2002).

Misconceptions are common. Many young people believe that women cannot become pregnant at sexual debut; that symptoms of infection go away on their own; that one can clearly identify an infected person by their appearance; that pregnancy can occur through physical embrace; or that infection is transmitted through everyday activities or can be prevented by proper personal hygiene (Brown et al., 2001). Among young women aged up to 24 years in India for example, while 37 per cent have heard of AIDS, only three in five could identify such risk factors as multiple partner relations (57 per cent) or irregular condom use (58 per cent). Also disturbing is that only one quarter (26 per cent) are aware that a healthy looking person could be HIV-positive (UNICEF, UNAIDS and WHO, 2002). Indeed, the National Behavioural Surveillance Survey reports that only 28 per cent of young men and 26 per cent of young women harbour no misconceptions about transmission (NACO and UNICEF, 2002). Indeed, the NACO National Behavioural Surveillance Survey reports that only 30 and 22 per cent, respectively, of urban and rural males aged 15-19 and 32 and 20 per cent, correspondingly, of young females harbour no misconceptions about the transmission of HIV (NACO and UNICEF, 2002). State-wise variations are evident. Correct awareness of three leading misconceptions—that mosquito bites and sharing a meal with an infected person do not transmit HIV/AIDS, and that a healthy looking person can transmit HIV/AIDS—was limited among adolescents in all states, but appears to be particularly limited among those residing in the northern and eastern states. Gender disparities remain narrow in each state.

Adolescents are poorly informed about the physiological changes associated with maturation (Joseph et al., 1997; UNESCO, 2000; VNESI, 1999). In school settings, where programmes on population, family life and sex education exist, they focus more on biological and scientific information than broader issues of sexuality (Chakrabarti, 2003). Young people are also unlikely to be aware of services available to them or of their right to avail these services. For example, adolescent abortion-seekers in Pune tended to believe that abortion services were not legally available to unmarried women (Ganatra and Hirve, 2002b). Gate-keeper attitudes ensure that young people remain poorly informed; gatekeepers typically (mis)-perceive that deliberate withholding or obfuscating of information are protective strategies.

Television, peers and erotic literature are by far the most commonly cited sources of information on sexual and reproductive matters although the information they provide is not always accurate. For example, among low-income college boys in Mumbai, erotic materials were the main source of information (Abraham, 2001). A study of adolescent girls aged 13-17 in Haryana reports that for almost all, the leading source of information was television (73 per cent) and/or radio (37 per cent) (Singh, Devi and Gupta, 1999). The NACO National Behavioural Surveillance Survey suggests that by and large, young people are relatively unexposed to the large range of media providing messages on HIV/AIDS: while 76 per cent were exposed to such messages on television, far fewer (between one-third and half) were exposed to messages through the radio or newspapers/magazines, and between 6 per cent and 12 per cent through billboards, pamphlets or films. In contrast, even fewer—about 15 per cent of males and females—were exposed to inter-personal communication on the topic (NACO and UNICEF, 2002).

Sensitive interventions have succeeded in raising awareness of risky behaviours and dispelling myths concerning protection among adolescent girls and boys (Awasthi, Nichter and Pande, 2000; Sebastian et al., 2002b). An intervention among adolescent girls in Allahabad reports that 94 per cent were able to name an STI at the midline compared to 67 per cent at the baseline; 98 per cent knew that pregnancy occurs through sexual contact whereas only 44 per cent knew this at the baseline (Sebastian et al., 2002b). Among adolescent boys in a Lucknow slum, exposure to an innovative education programme dramatically increased knowledge (Awasthi, Nichter and Pande, 2000). However as evidence from other settings warns, improved awareness by itself is insufficient in changing behaviour, but is only one of several necessary actions.

Limited self-efficacy, negotiation, life and livelihood skills

Gender double standards and power imbalances shape adolescents' lives and often undermine their ability to make informed sexual and reproductive choices both in marital and premarital partnerships. The high priority placed on preserving young women's chastity before marriage can constrain girls' education, access to services, age at marriage, autonomy and mobility. Young females have a limited voice in matters relating to their own lives—whether to continue schooling, decisions on when and whom to marry, physical mobility and sexual relations. Young men are affected by a different set of gender-based expectations, including social pressure to have sex at an early age, often under conditions that place them at risk of infection. Gender power imbalances are observed in both marital and premarital partnerships. In many cases, male partners, parents or in-laws play a leading role as decision makers.

Among the unmarried

A number of studies highlight the persistence of widespread gender-based double standards in India with regard to female chastity and premarital sexual activity. Adolescent girls are acutely aware of the restrictions that are imposed on them, whether on dress, speech or mobility. For example, girls may even be asked to discontinue attending school when they reach puberty, or not to go out alone (Mehra, Savithri and Coutinho, 2002). Arranged marriage and extensive dowries continue to characterise marriage across the country. Young women rarely have any say in marriage decisions; indeed, some are married early against their will at the behest of their parents.

Young people themselves often accept—and even justify—double standards that condone and even encourage premarital relations for men but not for women (Mehra, Savithri and Coutinho, 2002). Many young people feel that society condones premarital sexual activity among boys and even puts social pressure on boys to become sexually active at an early age (Mehra, Savithri and Coutinho, 2002; Sodhi and Verma, forthcoming).

Premarital sexual relations among adolescent girls are characterised by unequal power relations. Young women are much more likely than men to report love and commitment as leading reasons for engaging in sexual relations; the fear of losing a partner, incurring his anger or jeopardising the relationship are important factors inhibiting young women from exercising choice over whether and when to have sex and whether to use condoms (Sodhi and Verma, forthcoming).

Among the married

Within the age and gender-stratified family structure that characterises much of India, young, newly married women face major constraints on their autonomy in the marital home. The average adolescent bride is unlikely to have had a say on whether or not to have sexual relations, or when to bear children. On the contrary, society often places strong pressures on women to prove their fertility and, in many settings, bearing sons is the only means by which young women can establish social acceptance and economic security in their marital homes. Married girls often have limited access to health care or decision-making authority (Barua and Kurz, 2001; Kulkarni, 2003; Santhya and Jejeebhoy, 2003). Further analysis of NFHS data shows, for example, that although decision-making authority is limited among women in general, married adolescents are particularly unlikely to participate in household decisions, whether those relating to major purchases or their own health care. Age has been found to play a more powerful role in enhancing decision-making authority than other socio-demographic factors, including education (Santhya and Jejeebhoy, 2003).

There is emerging evidence, though limited, of young girls negotiating wanted outcomes and making decisions on whether to engage in a partnership, when and whom to marry and matters affecting their own lives (Mehra, Savithri and Coutinho, 2002). A recent study has documented increases in self-efficacy and autonomy among out-of-school adolescent girls who participated in a comprehensive education and service intervention. The intervention provided non-formal, family life and vocational education as well as service provision, opportunities to learn how to use banks and public transport, to participate in recreational activities and to receive leadership training. Those who participated in the programme were, for example, more likely to display autonomy and self-confidence, and more likely to make independent decisions, such as decisions on marriage (25 per cent vs. 7 per cent), and to have gone to a health centre alone (25 vs. 6 per cent) in the last six months. These differences in autonomy were significant even after controlling for education of girls and their parents. In terms of reproductive health-seeking behaviour, as Figure 5 suggests, those who had married in the interval (n=292) reported significantly more positive behaviours compared to married controls (n=269) in a host of indicators related to reproductive health and child survival: they were more likely to have married at age 18 or later, to use contraception and to have sought pregnancy-related care if they became pregnant (Levitt-Dayal et al., 2003).

Figure 5

Intervention participants and non-participants reporting selected reproductive health behaviours (%)

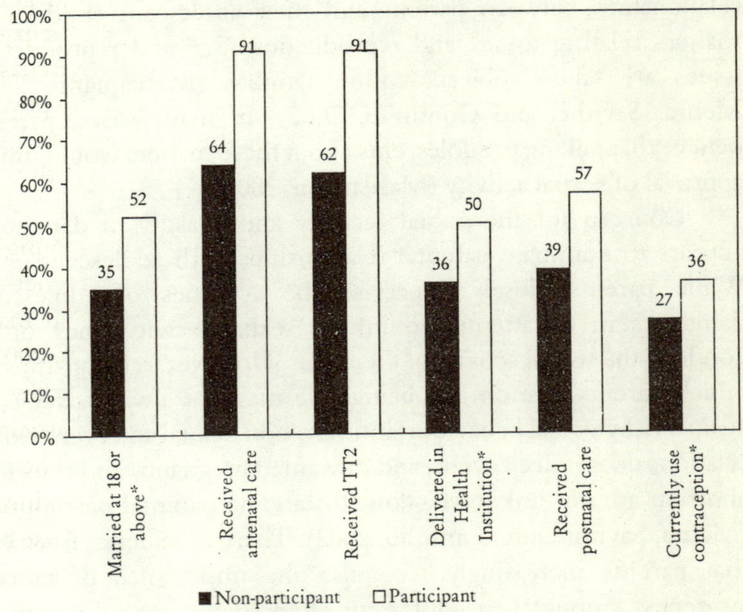

* Becomes non-significant when controlling for girls' education.

Source: Levitt-Dayal et al., 2003.

A number of programmes are available for girls in different parts of the country that attempt to build skills and livelihoods, provide training and education, or more generally, empower them in ways that may have a bearing on their sexual and reproductive health awareness and exercise of reproductive choices; for example, the Indira Soochana Shakti Yojana, the Balika Samriddhi Yojana, the Kishori Shakti Yojana, the Shagun scheme (Punjab) and the Gujarat Bicycle Scheme. Programmes operating under the ICDS scheme offer training in thrift, credit services, health and hygiene.

Limited communication, interaction and support on sexual and reproductive health matters

Lack of communication, interaction and support characterise relationships between parents and their adolescent children in matters relating to sex and reproduction. Sex and reproductive issues are taboo subjects within families (Masilamani, 2003; Mehra, Savithri and Coutinho, 2002). In many cases, parents believe that talking to adolescents about these matters would imply approval of sexual activity (Masilamani, 2003).

Concern for the sexual security and chastity of daughters appears to dominate parental relationships with adolescent girls. While parents closely supervise the activities of adolescent daughters in an attempt to inhibit sexual activity, they often condone the sexual activity of their sons. However, relationships in which parents take on a policing role may not always safeguard against risky sexual behaviour: intimate non-sexual and even sexual relations does indeed occur, and unwanted pregnancy and resort to abortion are not unknown, notwithstanding parental perceptions (Mehra, Savithri and Coutinho, 2002). There is evidence however that parents increasingly recognise the importance of raising awareness among their adolescent children but are inhibited by lack of in-depth knowledge and embarrassment to do this themselves (Damayanthi, 2003; Sebastian et al., 2003; Subba Rao, 2003).

Few studies have explored the links between parental support and protection from risk. Those that do hint that family support may be key in influencing safe sex behaviours. For example, a study of low-income college students in Mumbai reveals a positive relationship between perceived authoritarian family relationships and early sexual debut among young males (Abraham and Kumar, 1999). Another study of 16-year-old students in Goa suggests however that adolescents—especially girls—who experience unwanted sexual relations are more likely than others to report lack of communication and support in the relationship with their parents (Patel and Andrew, 2001). And a recent study of adolescent abortion-seekers suggests that fear of parents, fear of disclosure of pregnancy status and lack of perceived parental support may have led many pregnant adolescents to delay an abortion or to seek an abortion from unqualified providers (Ganatra and Hirve, 2002b).

Lack of youth-centred and youth-led programmes on sexual and reproductive health

Although there are a host of laws and programmes that seek to protect aspects of young people's sexual and reproductive health and ability to exercise their rights, these have rarely been implemented in ways that address the needs of adolescents, whether married or unmarried.

Though there is a law stipulating the minimum age at marriage, it is not strictly enforced. Large proportions of young women continue to marry and bear children in adolescence and exercise little autonomy over their sexual and reproductive lives. There are limited programmes that make concerted efforts to delay early marriage or address married adolescents as a distinct group. Hence, while the adverse consequences of pregnancy in adolescence are well known, adolescents are not more likely to receive antenatal or intra-partum care than adult women are (IIPS and ORC Macro, 2000; Santhya and Jejeebhoy, 2003). Almost one-third of adolescents who gave birth in the three years preceding NFHS 2 received no antenatal care; 31 per cent delivered in an institution and 42 per cent were delivered by a trained attendant. Of those delivering at home, only 18 per cent were followed up in the post-partum period. By and large it is the northern states in which pregnancy-related care of adolescents is particularly limited—in such states as Haryana, Rajasthan, Madhya Pradesh, Uttar Pradesh and Bihar for example, 40 per cent or more recently delivered adolescents had received no antenatal care, fewer than one-quarter had delivered in an institution, and fewer than one-third were delivered by a trained attendant. In contrast, in Punjab, and the western and southern states, considerably larger proportions have received pregnancy-related care—even so, care is by no means universal (IIPS and ORC Macro, 2000).

Few programmes attend to the needs of married young women for care of gynaecological disorders. For example, only 49 per cent of married young women who experienced a gynaecological problem in rural Maharashtra, India and 9 per cent of those experiencing RTI/STI symptoms in rural Tamil Nadu sought care (Joseph, Prasad and Abraham, 2003).

Access to abortion services is considerably more limited among young females compared to adult women, and is particularly poor among the unmarried. Evidence suggests that adolescents—particularly unmarried adolescents—are more likely than older women to seek abortions from unqualified or untrained providers, to have delayed abortions and undergo second trimester abortions, and to suffer complications. Lack of access to services and other resources are factors contributing to adolescents' reluctance to seek safe and early abortions on the one hand, and seek care in case of complications on the other. Unqualified or traditional providers are frequently preferred because they are perceived as providing prompt and anonymous care. There is evidence that, in some cases, providers charged unmarried women more for their services (Ganatra and Hirve, 2003).

While unmarried adolescents are technically eligible for all services offered to the married under the family welfare programme, in practice they have little access to these. Evidence suggests that adolescents want to know more about their bodies, about relationships, sex and reproduction; yet neither counselling, nor knowledge on sexuality reaches them. Unmarried adolescent abortion-seekers are more likely than other women to delay abortion beyond the first trimester and choose home remedies and unqualified providers (see for example, Ganatra and Hirve, 2002b). Findings of irregular use of contraceptives reported in studies of premarital sexual partnerships suggest that access to condoms and contraception is likewise limited (Abraham and Kumar, 1999).

As reflected in the NACO National Behavioural Surveillance Survey, care-seeking among this group of married and unmarried youth is not universal. Fewer than half of all young men and about one third of all young women sought medical care for their symptoms (NACO and UNICEF, 2002).

Factors impeding use of services by unmarried youth are poorly studied in India, but as in other settings are likely to include a range of provider- and facility-based obstacles—limited accessibility, high costs, lack of privacy and confidentiality, poor counselling skills, threatening provider attitudes and indifferent quality of care (Senderowitz, 1999).

While the need to provide 'accessible' and 'friendly' services to youth is acknowledged, there is less clarity about what these terms imply. It is evident that young people want access to confidential services without fear of discovery by family or community members; that are available at convenient locations and times, do not require long waits, are affordable, and most important, provided by staff who are non-threatening, non-judgmental and willing to respect confidentiality. There is some evidence that where anonymity is assured (e.g. telephone hotlines or the letter-box approach to communication and counselling), adolescents do take appropriate steps to obtain information. Interventions —for example 'youth friendly' services established in a dedicated space in a government hospital in New Delhi—have been implemented that will shed light on the extent to which adolescents access these services or perceive them as non-judgemental and confidential (Mehta, 2003). Lessons learned from a similar experience in Thailand suggest that hospital settings may not attract young people however friendly the services; rather there is a need to house services at more acceptable locations such as department stores, youth centres and colleges (Poonkhum, 2003). A study that sought the views of adolescent girls reports that girls did indeed express the need for a separate clinic for young people that would be served by female providers (Joseph et al., 1997).

Sangath's adolescent and family programme in Goa is one example of services provided to adolescents in a safe and private setting. Services are based on the recognition that educational needs, access to appropriate services and parental communication are key to healthy adolescence, and are delivered in ways that accommodate young people's stated priorities: "a welcoming facility, where I can drop in and be attended to quickly"; "where there is privacy and confidentiality," "where staff treat us with respect and do not judge us" (Godinho et al., 2002).

Changing policy and programme environment

Over the course of the 1990s, the policy environment has begun to shed its ambivalence on the need to address the sexual and reproductive health needs of young people. At the international level, the International Conference on Population and Development (ICPD) and ICPD+5 have reiterated the importance of providing information, counselling and services for youth, achieving universal access to primary education, closing the gender gap in primary and secondary school education; and, more generally, respecting the reproductive rights of adolescents and youth. Indeed, by 1999, the recommendations of ICPD+5 included the recognition of young people's vulnerability to HIV and recommended attention to reducing prevalence in this age group. Other notable conventions ratified by India that have implications for addressing the reproductive and sexual rights of young people include, most notably, the Convention on the Rights of the Child (CRC) and the Convention on the Elimination of All Forms of Discrimination Against Women (CEDAW).

At the national level, these commitments to meeting young people's sexual and reproductive health needs and rights have been acknowledged. The National Population Policy, 2000 recognises, for the first time, that adolescents constitute an under-served group with special sexual and reproductive health needs that have remained unmet. The Policy advocates special programmatic attention to delay marital age, provide free and compulsory education up to the age of 14 and provide nutritional services. It specifically recommends the need to "ensure for adolescents access to information, counselling and services, including reproductive health services, that are affordable and accessible," and to "strengthen primary health centres and sub-centres to provide counselling, both to adolescents and also to newly weds" (MOHFW, 2000).

The recognition of the spread of the HIV/AIDS epidemic among young people has resulted in a greater openness in addressing issues relating to sex among young people. The National AIDS Policy, 2000, for example, focuses on the population between 18 and 40 years, and discusses more directly, measures to address risky sexual behaviour, although it does not identify adolescents as a special group.

The draft National Youth Policy, 2000 addresses the needs of those aged 13 to 35. It stresses the need for a multi-sectoral approach to youth, with a focus on 'youth empowerment,' notably education, skills building and leadership as well as nutrition and equal opportunity. While it discusses the need for access to health services among young people, particularly women, and cites the need for reproductive health "guidance," population and family life education, its primary focus is nutrition and education rather than sexual and reproductive health.

In connection with the preparation of the Tenth Five-year Plan (2002-07), a working group for the Welfare and Development of Adolescents was established to provide input into the Plan. Its report makes recommendations pertaining to all aspects of adolescent life. It notes the need for more meaningful education (formal and non-formal, life skills and livelihood training). It advocates changes in the conditions of working adolescents and attention to the kinds of work that adolescents "can and cannot" do. It stresses gender issues and the different needs of boys and girls. It highlights the health and nutrition needs of adolescents and the need for counselling, a supportive environment and youth participation in development planning. Finally, it pays attention to issues of national integration, and sports and adventure, and notes the needs of adolescents in difficult circumstances. The Working Group advocated that the most appropriate location for issues of adolescence is the Ministry of Youth Affairs and Sports, but recognised the need to substantially strengthen this Ministry to expand its mandate to address adolescents in a meaningful way. It recommended moreover a decentralised approach focused on municipal, taluka and panchayat levels (Planning Commission, 2001).

Several programmes have been undertaken at the national level that translate the recommendations of these policies into action. The Reproductive and Child Health Programme, whose second phase is about to be launched, made a paradigm shift in the mid-1990s, from contraceptive targets to a client-centred focus on health needs, better quality gender-sensitive information and services, and ensuring access. While the programme recognises that youth are a special population with special needs, specific measures to ensure their sexual and reproductive health and rights have not yet been advocated.

The Ministry of Youth Affairs and Sports undertakes programmes, under the broad umbrella of the Nehru Yuvak Kendras, to raise health awareness and adopt health-promoting practices, particularly with regard to issues relating to sexual and reproductive health. Activities also include the development of livelihood skills and training in self-employment. Programmes are being implemented unevenly across states (see for example the assessment of the Working Group for the Welfare and Development of Adolescents, Planning Commission, 2001).

At the state level, a number of innovations have been initiated. Several states have introduced specific programmes for youth, including in school and community settings. For example, in Andhra Pradesh, the Education Department launched a successful four-day AIDS education programme with a life skills focus in school settings. The programme experience concluded that adult gatekeepers—parents and teachers in particular—may pose a significant challenge in promoting school-based awareness. There was considerable demand for the programme among young people, which was perceived by them to be an appropriate mechanism through which sexual and reproductive health awareness can be imparted. Considerable demand for an extension of such programmes has been generated both among students and out-of-school youth (Damayanthi, 2003).

A number of programmes in different parts of the country do not focus directly on the sexual and reproductive health of young people, notably girls, but attempt to build skills and livelihoods, provide training and education, or more generally, empower girls in ways that may have a bearing on their sexual and reproductive health awareness and exercise of reproductive choices. For example, the Indira Soochana Shakti Yojana, the Balika Samriddhi Yojana, the Kishori Shakti Yojana, the Shagun Scheme (Punjab), and schemes operating under the Integrated Child Development Services (ICDS) programme offer girls training in thrift, credit services, health, hygiene and so on. Other schemes—notably the Apni Beti, Apna Dhan scheme and the Rajalakshmi scheme of Unit Trust of India—offer families monetary incentives for delaying the marriage age of their daughters beyond 18 years; under these schemes, insurance policies are drawn up in the girl's name and mature in her name if she has not married by age 18. While an array of schemes exist, however, they have a limited reach, and have rarely been evaluated.

The way forward

An increasing number of young people are experiencing risky or unwanted sexual activity resulting in adverse reproductive health outcomes for which they do not receive prompt or appropriate care. Contextual factors such as poverty, gender imbalances and lack of education or livelihood opportunities exacerbate their vulnerability. These are compounded by factors at the family, community and facility level. Much of their knowledge of sexual and reproductive health is superficial and lack of communication with parents and other trusted adults keeps young people ill informed. Education on sexuality remains inadequate and irrelevant to young people's needs, and services remain inaccessible, unacceptable, unaffordable and of indifferent quality.

While sexual and reproductive health needs of adolescents and young people are firmly on the national agenda, much remains to be done before programmes can be said to have responded to meeting their needs. Young people are a heterogeneous group whose situation, vulnerabilities, strengths and needs vary greatly, and policies and programmes will have to address these diverse needs through a multi-sectoral approach. While the voice of young people is key in programme design, implementation and evaluation, successful interventions will have to involve a wide constituency—including parents, teachers and religious and community leaders.

Programme recommendations

- Young people need to be equipped with knowledge and information on diverse issues, ranging from risk and protective sexual behaviours, including the role of condoms, to physical maturation, formation of partnerships, sources of information, counselling and services, their rights in accessing services and exercising choices. Sex and family life education must be imparted in ways that meet the needs of those in and out-of-school, responding to, rather than obfuscating, their sexual health questions.
- Equally important is the acquisition of life skills that will enable youth to put information into practice, encourage them to break down gender stereotypes and relate to each other as equals, develop self-esteem, as well as strengthen their abilities in problem-solving, decision-making, communication and inter-personal relations and negotiation.
- Parents, teachers and the adult community must facilitate and be involved in this process, whether through free and open communication, or by creating environments that protect adolescents from abuse, and enable them to access information and the full range of services. Programmes are needed at the family and community levels that enable parents and other community members to overcome their discomfort, enhance their knowledge of adolescent health and development, and improve their communication skills. Programmes are also needed that convince parents of the need

to focus on enhancing informed choice among adolescents rather than imposing close supervision and controls as a more effective strategy of ensuring sexual and reproductive well-being.

- Messages on the legal age at marriage, the adverse consequences of early marriage, and the importance of eliminating gender double standards and imbalances that may adversely affect the lives of both boys and girls must be reinforced.
- Girls and boys, married and unmarried have different priorities and needs, and must overcome a different set of obstacles in accessing sexual and reproductive health information and services. In order to be 'youth-friendly,' programmes and services must recognise that young people's needs and lives are different from those of children and adults, and respect these needs in an acceptable and non-threatening manner. The involvement of youth in adapting programmes—design, implementation, monitoring and evaluating—is essential.

Research recommendations

This review highlights the huge gaps in knowledge that remain. To make informed policy decisions, we need more social science and operations research to understand how the situation and needs of different groups of adolescents—married and unmarried, girls and boys, older and younger. Equally, we need to better understand whether and why their sexual and reproductive health needs remain unmet, why informed choice continues to elude them and how services should be structured to overcome the social, cultural and economic constraints they face.

- Young people are facing a changing social environment in the context of rapid globalisation and the increasing impact of the media and information technology on the one hand, and growing fundamentalism on the other, which have led to a questioning of traditional norms and behaviours. Research is needed that explores how these influence young people and how they can make a transition to safe sexual lives in a new and changing context.

- The patterns of formation and conduct of sexual partnerships among young people remain an important, unexplored area of research. Questions that need attention include: What are the nature and duration of different types of partnerships? Do females and males have different perceptions or expectations of relationships? How do females and males perceive sexual responsibility or 'appropriate' behaviour within relationships? How do expectations of a relationship influence decisions to practice contraception or safe sex? And to what extent, and by whom, are choices exercised regarding sexual behaviour and the avoidance of disease and unwanted pregnancy? Given increasing HIV among youth, it is critical that research explores the context of risky early sexual encounters and the obstacles youth face in practicing safer sex.
- Findings confirm that for the majority of sexually active girls, sexual activity is initiated within the context of marriage. Research is needed that articulates the manifold needs of married adolescents—for information, for skills in articulating and negotiating safe and wanted sexual and reproductive health outcomes, and exercising greater autonomy in these matters. Equally, what is needed is operations research that will test the feasibility and acceptability of integrated health and social interventions that would increase young females' reproductive health knowledge and practices, and ability to act in their own interests.
- Research is needed that explores the ways in which gender roles/expectations and power imbalances in family structures limit or affect life skills among young females and males. More specifically, research is needed to examine ways in which gender double standards and resulting behaviour compromises sexual and reproductive health among females and males—with regard to risk behaviours, the timing of marriage, or choices regarding parenthood. Of interest in many settings is research that explores the constraints that

married adolescent and young women face in accessing information and services, in influencing decisions about fertility, contraception, morbidity and sexual relations, and in remaining safe from disease, violence and unwanted pregnancy. Research is also needed that identifies circumstances under which adolescent and young women may be able to exercise greater autonomy in these matters.

- Available evidence suggests that significant minorities of sexually active young males and even females experience infection and unintended pregnancy, yet little is known about the pathways they follow in treating the infection or resolving the pregnancy. Community-based studies are needed that reveal patterns of infection experienced by youth, and their socio-economic and behavioural correlates including the role of condoms. For females, moreover, research is needed that explores abortion behaviour among both unmarried and married adolescent girls, the decision making process, and factors that underlie delays in seeking termination, resort to untrained providers and higher rates of complications among unmarried young women.
- Young people, especially females, are observed to be particularly vulnerable to sexual coercion and violence. Sometimes this coercion clearly involves the use of force, at other times it is subtler and involves economic or psychological manipulation. A considerable amount of further research is needed that sensitively explores the levels, patterns, nature and extent of sexual coercion and violence. Another question that must be answered is that of how the presence or threat of violence/coercion limits the ability of young people to negotiate safe sex and/or contraception, their ability to make reproductive choices, and their ability generally to influence their own reproductive and sexual health.
- Research is needed that explores the use of sexual and reproductive health services by youth and the socio-cultural and programme-related constraints they face in doing so. What is available suggests that few services in fact exist which cater to

their special health and information needs. Likewise, there are few opportunities for adolescents to seek information or counselling on sexual and reproductive matters. It is critical that research documents young people's own perceptions and priorities with regard to appropriate and acceptable delivery mechanisms for sexual and reproductive health services.

- Much of our research has tended to focus on risk behaviours and their determinants. Yet, findings have pointed to a number of actions that protect. There is a need for in-depth studies to substantiate or provide greater insight into these protective pathways, and to provide a stronger evidence base on protective actions and strategies for different groups of young people.
- There are an increasing number of programmes for youth intended to raise awareness, build self-efficacy or provide friendly services. However, these models remain poorly tested and we know little about their feasibility, acceptability, effectiveness and replicability. Research is needed that provides evidence-based directions for future programming.

Domestic Violence

Vijaya Nidadavolu

Violence against women is both a human rights issue as well as a public health concern as it impacts women's reproductive, sexual and mental health. Evidence reveals that women in India experience violence in various forms throughout their lives, and it cuts across boundaries of caste, class, region and religion.

Prevalence of physical, emotional and sexual violence

Domestic violence is a complex issue to research as the extent and forms of its occurrence remain largely hidden and there is a great degree of social acceptance of the issue. Data should be interpreted carefully as women often under-report violence out of a feeling of shame or because they do not view certain acts as violent (IIPS and ORC Macro, 2000; INCLEN, 2000; Jejeebhoy, 1998b).

According to NFHS 2, 21 per cent of ever-married women in India have been physically mistreated by their husbands, in-laws or other persons since age 15; 19 per cent have been beaten by their husbands and 11 per cent had been beaten in the 12 months prior to the study (IIPS and ORC Macro, 2000). While National Crimes Records Bureau figures reveal an increase in reporting of gender-based violence from 31 per cent in 1995 to 45 per cent in

1999 (NCRB, 1995-99), evidence is also emerging from population-based surveys suggesting that between 21 to 48 per cent of women from different socio-cultural settings in India have experienced physical violence (INCLEN, 2000; Jejeebhoy, 1998b; Verma and Collumbien, 2003; Visaria, 1999b). These estimates are corroborated by studies investigating reporting patterns of men, with 21-40 per cent of men in different studies reporting perpetrating physical violence (Duvvury, Nayak and Allendorf, 2002; Martin et al., 1999; Verma and Collumbien, 2003). Estimates from facility-based surveys, such as hospitals, courts, NGOs and police records, reflect similar prevalence rates (Daga, Jejeebhoy and Rajgopal, 1998; Jaswal, 2000).

A closer scrutiny of the prevalence rates reveals some state-wise variation. Tamil Nadu shows the highest prevalence, with 40 per cent of the women reporting experiencing physical violence since age 15. Andhra Pradesh, Karnataka, Meghalaya, Arunachal Pradesh, Mizoram, Orissa, Bihar and Jammu and Kashmir have prevalence rates higher than 20 per cent. Himachal Pradesh shows the lowest prevalence rate at 5.8 per cent, followed by Kerala (10.1 per cent) and Gujarat (10.2 per cent) (IIPS and ORC Macro, 2000). An examination of the National Crimes Records Bureau statistics reveals that reporting of crimes against women at home, or cruelty by husband and his relatives, are higher is states like Kerala (80 cases per million population) and Gujarat (82 cases per million population) (NCRB, 1995-99). While it is difficult to draw definite conclusions from data about the state-wise variation, it can be clearly said that domestic violence is a country-wide phenomena.

Evidence on emotional violence is limited, with few studies enquiring about its incidence. Findings suggest that emotional violence ranges from rates of 23 per cent (Visaria, 1999b) to 27 per cent (Jejeebhoy, 1998b), 43 per cent (INCLEN, 2000) and 72 per cent (Duvvury, Nayak and Allendorf, 2002).

Evidence on sexual violence, as in the case of emotional violence, is limited. The INCLEN study reveals that 15 per cent of the total sample of women reported one or more incidents of forced sex during the 12 months prior to the study (INCLEN, 2000). In a study in Kheda district, Gujarat, 20 per cent of the women reporting physical violence described abuse of a sexual nature (Visaria, 1999b). Studies with men reveal between 29 per cent (Martin et al., 1999) and 50 per cent (Duvvury, Nayak and Allendorf, 2002) reporting perpetrating sexual violence.

Domestic violence is rarely an isolated event. In a study of 4,005 women reporting physical violence, 63 per cent reported the experience more than three times (INCLEN, 2000). A study of men indicates that 50 per cent reported perpetrating sexual violence, of whom 39 per cent reported perpetrating violence more than ten times in the 12 months prior to the study (Duvvury, Nayak and Allendorf, 2002).

Correlates of domestic violence

Evidence on the factors underlying the experience of domestic violence among women suggests that socio-demographic factors and, more consistently, gender norms and power imbalances continue to justify and perpetuate its occurrence.

Socio-demographic factors

Although domestic violence affects women of all classes, ages, religious groups and castes, socio-demographic variations are observed. NFHS 2 evidence suggests that more recently married women (those who have married within the past 5 years) are less likely to have suffered violence than women married for longer durations (14 per cent vs 21-23 per cent), but this may be a reflection of the fact that women married for a shorter duration are less exposed to such episodes. Studies also suggest that women residing in nuclear households may be more likely to experience domestic violence than women in joint families (IIPS and ORC Macro, 2000; Jejeebhoy, 1998b; Visaria, 1999b).

While better-off women are generally less likely to report an experience than other women (IIPS and ORC Macro, 2000; INCLEN, 2000), this variation should be interpreted cautiously as women who are better educated and from a higher income group may be less likely than others to disclose such experiences (INCLEN, 2000). Findings from NFHS 2 also suggest that women residing in urban areas are less likely to report the experience of violence than those residing in rural areas (17 per cent and 23 per cent, respectively). Educational disparities are even wider: women with no education (26 per cent) are three times more likely to experience beatings than women who have completed high school (9 per cent) (IIPS and ORC Macro, 2000). Other authors speculate that there may be a transition and women who have begun to exert their autonomy—the urban, better educated and economically active, for example—may in fact suffer more violence than other women precisely because of the greater agency they exert in their own lives, thereby challenging existing gender norms (Jejeebhoy, 1998b; INCLEN, 2000).

Gender norms and power imbalances

There is considerable evidence that domestic violence against women is widely accepted and justified in India, and perceived by both women and men as normal in married life (Duvvury, Nayak and Allendorf, 2002; IIPS and ORC Macro, 2000; INCLEN, 2000; Jejeebhoy, 1998b). Studies have inquired into the justification of wife-beating under a variety of circumstances, ranging from disobedience and disrespect to in-laws, to infidelity and alcohol abuse. As seen in Figure 6, among the most persistent circumstances in which violence is justified by women are those related to perceptions of non-performance of domestic duties or non-compliance with expectations (IIPS and ORC Macro, 2000; INCLEN, 2000; Jejeebhoy, 1998b; Visaria, 1999b).

Evidence suggests some variation in responses. NFHS 2 findings show for example that 40 per cent of women justify violence if a wife neglects the house or children, but only 7 per cent justify it if the wife's natal family did not comply with the husband's demands for money or jewellery. Better educated and urban women are less likely to justify wife beating than are other

Figure 6

Ever-married women who agree with specific reasons for justifying a husband beating his wife, 1998-99 (%)

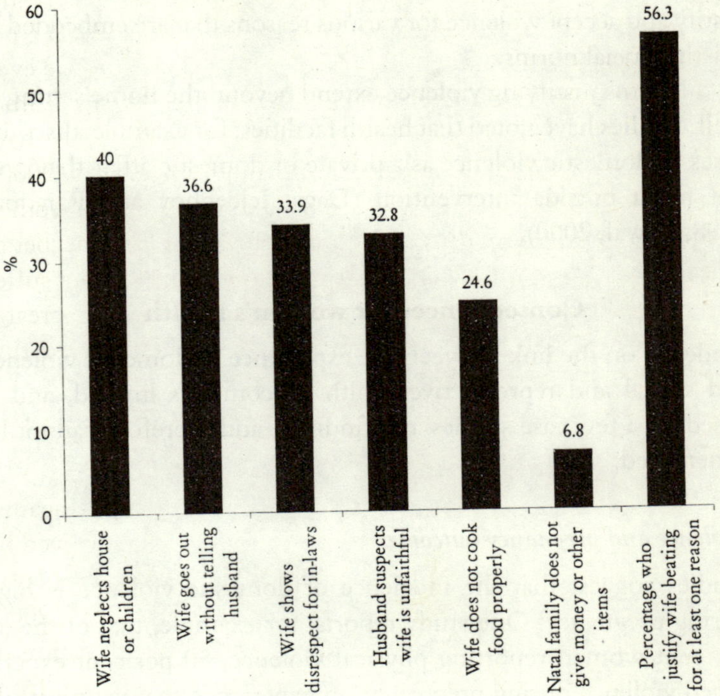

Source: IIPS and ORC Macro, 2000.

women. Adolescents aged 15-19 years—presumably comprising those with least autonomy—are more likely to justify violence than older women (IIPS and ORC Macro, 2000).

Findings of studies of men suggest that men justify wife-beating for similar reasons. In a study in Uttar Pradesh, almost two-thirds of the men felt that wives should follow the instructions of her husband and one in every four felt that physical violence was justified if the wife disobeyed the husband (EVALUATION Project, 1997). In another study, men agreed that violence is justified if the wife is sexually unfaithful (79 per cent), disrespectful to family elders (77 per cent) and disrespectful to the husband (75 per cent) (Duvvury, Nayak and Allendorf, 2002). In short, evidence points to the fact that men and women in India justify and accept violence for various reasons that are embedded in existing social norms.

Norms justifying violence extend beyond the home setting as well. Studies have noted that health facilities, for example, discount cases of domestic violence as a private or domestic affair that does not merit outside intervention (Daga, Jejeebhoy and Rajgopal, 1998; Jaswal, 2000).

Consequences for women's health

Evidence on the link between the experience of domestic violence and sexual and reproductive health outcomes is limited, and is based on a few case studies and findings, and therefore cannot be generalised.

Violence and pregnancy outcomes

Studies suggest that the incidence of domestic violence is high during pregnancy. One study reports, for example, that of the 40 per cent women reporting physical violence, 50 per cent experienced violence during pregnancy, an experience that is uniformly reported by women across all socio-economic strata (INCLEN, 2000).

There is evidence of an association between the experience of violence during pregnancy and mortality. For example, a study of maternal mortality that explored, in depth, causes of 121 maternal death reports that the second largest cause of deaths in pregnancy (nearly 16 per cent) resulted from complications associated with the experience of domestic violence (Ganatra, Coyaji and Rao, 1998). Foetal and infant deaths have also been associated with the experience of domestic violence during pregnancy (Jejeebhoy, 1998a; Ramasubban and Rishyasringa, 1998).

Violence and symptoms of reproductive tract infections or sexually transmitted infections

The link between perpetration of violence and experience of symptoms of infection has been observed. Studies have hypothesised that women who suffer physical violence are less likely to be in a position to negotiate safe sex or condom use with their husbands. There is also evidence that men who admit perpetrating violence on their wives also admit multiple partner sexual relations and non-use of condoms (Verma and Collumbien, 2003). Data reveal that abusive men are more likely to engage in extra-marital sex and have symptoms of STIs, thereby placing their wives at risk of acquiring infection (Martin et al., 1999; Verma and Collumbien, 2003).

Mental health outcomes

Evidence on the links of violence to mental ill-health in India is limited but studies from other countries suggest that perhaps the most long-lasting and persistent effects of violence are such mental health outcomes as depression and post-traumatic stress disorder, as well as sexual dysfunction and suicidal behaviour (Patel, 2002).

Violence, injury and related treatment-seeking

Studies have underscored that injuries resulting from domestic violence are widespread and severe. A multi-site study reports that almost half (45.3 per cent) of women who faced violence reported injuries that required treatment, and only half these women reported receiving health care. Of these, 23.5 per cent required treatment on more than five separate occasions, and 187 women out of a sample of 9,938 required hospitalisation as a result of their injuries (INCLEN, 2000). A similar study in Gujarat found that only 10 per cent reported requiring medical attention for injuries, and only 38 per cent of these women actually sought treatment (Visaria, 1999b).

The main reasons underlying women's reluctance to seek care relate to gender norms and power imbalances, embarrassment and shame, preference for relying on home remedies, and lack of control over economic resources required to seek care (INCLEN, 2000).

Women's inability to seek redress at the health system level is compounded by provider attitudes and skills. Many health care providers do not recognise a case of domestic violence, are not trained to assess or probe suspicious injuries in a sensitive manner, and consequently opportunities to identify and provide support to battered women are lost. This lack of skill and sensitivity is reflected in under-reporting of domestic violence in facility records and reports, and in treating and managing such cases (Jaswal, 2000).

The government's response

Laws, policies and programmes of the government have increasingly acknowledged the pervasiveness of domestic violence. A number of policy commitments and initiatives exist to tackle the health consequences of domestic violence, though there may not be a direct reference to recognising or addressing the issue (National Population Policy, 2000, Reproductive and Child Health Programme) (MOHFW, 1997). In contrast, the National Policy for the Empowerment of Women (MHRD, 2001) directly addresses domestic violence and makes commitments to set up institutions and mechanisms to assist women and increase their access to comprehensive, affordable and quality health care.

Legal responses are more direct. Section 498 A, IPC offers protection for women against cruelty in the home and against dowry demands. It provides that "whoever being the husband or the relative of the husband of a woman, subjects the woman to cruelty shall be punished for a term which may extend to 3 years and shall also be liable to fine". Cruelty is defined as "any wilful conduct which is of such a nature as is likely to drive the woman to commit suicide or to cause grave injury or danger to life, limb or health (whether physical or mental) of the woman". The law only takes cognisance of severe cases of domestic violence and not episodes that are less severe but which can have grave consequences.

The Ministry of Human Resource Development has circulated the draft Protection from Domestic Violence Bill, 2001, which is to be introduced in the Monsoon Session of Parliament in 2003. However, the Bill has several ambiguities and lacunae. The Bill recognises only those acts that are habitual in nature and cause misery as falling under domestic violence. Hence, there is no clear-cut assessment of other forms of violence, and such incidents remain open to interpretation by the judiciary (Lawyer's Collective, 2002).

Women's groups have noted the need instead for a civil law that recognises all forms of violence, including emotional, physical and sexual, and which gives women the right of residence in the marital home. They have also noted the need to recognise that any act of violence, rather than only habitual forms of violence, is recognised by the Bill.

The way ahead

Evidence on domestic violence remains sparse. Available studies suggest that domestic violence is pervasive and deeply rooted in socio-cultural norms. Women's lack of control over economic resources offers those facing violence few realistic options and a limited course of action. The police and the legal system are rarely accessed as there is little hope of redress.

Although disturbing proportions of women experience violence, programmes and laws have not been sensitive and redress continues to be limited. The state's response, in terms of health service provision, access to the police and legal opportunities are, in effect, limited. Community norms justifying domestic violence and social acceptance needs to be addressed through programme and research responses.

Programme recommendations

- It is important to advocate for a law that covers all forms of violence and offers women protection. While a progressive law can go a long way in giving succour to women it is also important that the entire judiciary is sensitised to the issue of domestic violence and is trained to deal with it.
- Programmes are needed that enhance women's autonomy, build life skills and provide livelihood opportunities so that they can develop self-confidence and exert greater agency over their own lives.
- Coordination is required between various government programmes, and interventions should involve existing local institutions such as panchayat bodies, self-help groups and neighbourhood committees. These institutions should be empowered to act as vigilance centres and to respond to cases of domestic violence to meet the health needs of women by linking them to services.
- Though men are the perpetrators of domestic violence, few interventions have actually worked to apprise men of women's (and their own) rights, raise male responsibility or involve men in family well-being. Interventions are required that work with men to sensitise them to the issue and devise long-term strategies to reduce the prevalence of violence.
- Screening protocols are required at primary, secondary and tertiary level health centres to identify cases of domestic violence. Health provider training must be reoriented to enable prompt recognition, sensitive probing, and appropriate counselling, treatment and referral for battered women. Concurrently, recording and reporting procedures used by hospitals and other health facilities need to be improved so that cases of violence are not 'lost'. Hospitals outside the government machinery also need to be encouraged to adopt similar screening protocols.
- It is important to set up linkages between health centres and other facilities such as the police and the law so that a

coordinated response is put in place. Health centres also need to be accessible and within the reach of women who are facing domestic violence.

Research recommendations

- Research is required that identifies factors that may be important in protecting women from domestic violence at the individual, family and community level on the one hand, and at the health service, police and legal system level on the other.
- While the few available studies have focused on the prevalence and correlates of domestic violence, little attention has been focused on the course of action women pursue and the obstacles they face when confronted with a situation of violence. A number of questions need to be addressed. For instance, what are the factors underlying inaction? In cases where women considered acting or did act, what measures were taken, how much support was available at the family and community levels, and how responsive were state mechanisms? These questions would shed light on the design of programmes intended to address battered women's needs, including those that focus on building self-efficacy, and life and livelihood skills.
- Few studies have documented the health consequences of domestic violence. Not only do we require research on a larger scale that explores reproductive morbidity, injuries and symptoms of RTIs/STIs but equally important are the mental health consequences of violence. At the same time, few studies have addressed such central issues of women's lives as economic and social conditions and support, and the ability to seek care for general health problems when women face severe violence at home.

Part III

Looking Back, Looking Forward

Looking Back, Looking Forward

Shireen J. Jejeebhoy and K.G. Santhya

Until a decade ago, policy makers, programme implementers and researchers paid little attention to broad sexual and reproductive health issues in India beyond that of family planning. The evidence compiled in this book suggests that in the last decade there has been a significant shift acknowledging the broad spectrum of sexual and reproductive health issues and the need for the exercise of reproductive rights, as well as a recognition that this change in focus has been long overdue.

A vast shift in orientation is evident in a number of policy documents and programmes. The National Population Policy, the Tenth Five-year Plan and the Reproductive and Child Health Programme, for example, all stand testimony to the fact that there is a commitment at the highest level to the broader health agenda. Unfortunately, there has been a huge schism between the articulation of and commitment to the new paradigm at the highest levels and its operationalisation at the community and grassroots level. Indeed, some states have deliberately opted not to embrace the wider concept of health.

The rights-based approach articulated in the National Population Policy has not yet filtered down to communities and women. The promotion of these rights is of particular relevance in the context of globalisation and its potential for excluding and marginalising the most vulnerable; yet we observe that the exercise of reproductive rights and informed sexual and reproductive choice continues to elude the most vulnerable and is still not reflected in the policies adopted by a number of state governments. Neither health sector reforms nor the service environment can be said to have fully implemented the rights-based approach.

Several services included in the expanded programme are, in reality, not yet accessible: for example, safe abortion and infertility services, contraception for the young, and even services for the management of infection and pregnancy. Despite the rapid spread of HIV/AIDS, programmes and policies tend to be cautious in their prevention focus. And while recent programmes have recognised the need to enhance quality of care elements, this has not been translated into reality.

Times are changing and there is a need for programmes to recognise this. The HIV pandemic has brought risky sexual behaviour to the forefront of sexual and reproductive health and programmes need to shed their traditional ambivalence and confront head-on such issues as premarital and extra-marital sex, appropriate counselling and accessible condom distribution. The special needs of young people must be recognised and the myth that informing young people about sexual matters makes them more likely to take risks disavowed. The disturbing misuse of new technologies, moreover, must be tackled—notable among these are the continued misuse of prenatal diagnostic techniques for sex-selective abortions, and poorly regulated and potentially exploitative access to ARTs. In short, new challenges have emerged and will undoubtedly continue to surface with regard to sexual and reproductive health issues, and programmes must be flexible and responsive to adapt to these needs.

Evidence on sexual and reproductive health information, services, behaviour and choice has expanded and become more in-depth, addressing subjects that were of limited interest a decade ago. Today, evidence is available on a multiplicity of issues, including women's rights and autonomy, and such sensitive issues as risky and premarital sexual relations, resort to sex-selective abortion and such programmatic themes as access to and quality of services. However, there continue to be gaps in what we know. Much of the information that is available comes, for example, from small studies that may not be generalisable. While the taboo surrounding investigation of sensitive behaviours may have been broken, far more evidence is required that highlights the factors underlying the persistence of unsafe or unwanted outcomes, notably those that have implications for the design of programmes. There is also a dearth of research that explores the feasibility, acceptability and replicability of intervention models intended to advance reproductive health and choice.

The agenda is challenging. However, there are encouraging signs of commitment to fulfilling this ambitious agenda. For one, the national commitment to the principles espoused in the ICPD Programme of Action and the National Population Policy remains firm. Sexual and reproductive health needs are clearly on the national agenda. There are, moreover, a growing number of programmes that appear to respond successfully to sexual and reproductive health needs in innovative and acceptable ways. And there are signs that civil society itself will hold governments accountable for implementing its commitments.

Bibliography

Abraham, L. 1997. Understanding youth sexuality: A study of college students in Mumbai. Summary report. Mumbai: Tata Institute of Social Sciences.

Abraham, L. 2001. Redrawing the *lakshman rekha*: Gender differences and cultural constructions in youth sexuality in urban India. *South Asia,* 24: 133-56.

Abraham, L. and K.A. Kumar. 1999. Sexual experiences and their correlates among college students in Mumbai city, India. *International Family Planning Perspectives*, 25(3): 139-46.

Acharya, R. and S. Sureender. 1996. Inter-spouse communication, contraceptive use and family size: Relationship examined in Bihar and Tamil Nadu. *Journal of Family Welfare,* 42(4): 5-11.

Aggarwal, A.K., R. Kumar, V. Gupta et al. 1999. Community-based study of reproductive tract infections among ever married women of reproductive age in a rural area of Haryana, India. *Journal of Communicable Diseases*, 31(4): 223-28.

Ahmed, S.I. 1992. Truck drivers as a vulnerable group in north east India. Paper presented at the 2nd International Congress on AIDS in Asia and the Pacific, New Delhi, 8-12 November.

AIDS Prevention and Control Project (APAC). 1998a. *Community Prevalence of Sexually Transmitted Diseases in Tamil Nadu 1998: A Report.* Chennai: APAC, Voluntary Health Services.

AIDS Prevention and Control Project (APAC). 1998b. *Realities of Sexual Behaviour in Tamil Nadu: A Report.* Chennai: APAC, Voluntary Health Services.

AIDS Prevention and Control Project (APAC). 1999. *STD Health Care Providers Survey in Tamil Nadu: A Report.* Chennai: APAC, Voluntary Health Services.

AIDS Prevention and Control Project (APAC). 2001. *HIV Risk Behaviour Surveillance Survey in Tamil Nadu: Report on Fifth Wave.* Chennai: APAC, Voluntary Health Services.

Andrew, G. and V. Patel. 2002. *Health Needs of Adolescents: A Study of Health Needs of Adolescents in Higher Secondary Schools in Goa.* Alto-Porvorim: Resource Centre for Adolescent and Child Health.

Anonymous. 2001. Despite efforts, maternal deaths in India remain common. *Population Briefs*, 7(3): 3.

Aras, R., N. Pai and A. Purandare. 1990. Perinatal mortality: A retrospective hospital study. *Journal of Obstetrics and Gynaecology,* 40(3): 365-69.

Aras, R., N. Pai, A. Baliga et al. 1989. Pregnancy at teenage: Risk factor for lower birth weight. *Indian Paediatrics,* 26(8): 823-25.

Arnold, F., S. Kishor and T.K. Roy. 2002. Sex selective abortions in India. *Population and Development Review*, 28(4): 759-86.

Asthana, S. and R. Oostvogels. 1996. Community participation in HIV prevention: Problems and prospects for community-based strategies among female sex workers in Madras. *Social Science and Medicine*, 43(2): 133-48.

Awasthi, S. and V.K. Pande. 1998. Sexual behaviour patterns and knowledge of sexually transmitted diseases in adolescent boys in urban slums of Lucknow. *Indian Paediatrics,* 35(11): 1105-9.

Awasthi, S., M. Nichter and V.K. Pande. 2000. Developing an interactive STD prevention programme for youth: Lessons from a north Indian slum. *Studies in Family Planning*, 31(2): 138-50.

Balaiah, D., D.D. Naik, R.C. Parida et al. 1999. Contraceptive knowledge, attitude and practices of men in rural Maharashtra. *Advances in Contraception*, 15: 217-34.

Bang, R. and A. Bang. 1994. Women's perception of white vaginal discharge: Ethnographic data from rural Maharashtra. In J. Gittleson et al., eds., *Listening to Women Talk about Their Health: Issues and Evidence from India*: 79-94. New Delhi: Har-Anand Publications.

Bang, R.A., A.T. Bang, M. Baitule et al. 1989. High prevalence of gynaecological diseases in rural Indian women. *Lancet*, 1(8629): 85-88.

Bang, A.T., R.A Bang, S. Baitule et al. 1999. Effect of home-based neonatal care and management of sepsis on neonatal mortality: Field trial in rural India. *Lancet*, 4, 354(9194): 1955-61.

Bang, A.T., R.A Bang, S. Baitule et al. 2001. Burden of morbidities and the unmet need for health care in rural neonates: A prospective observational study in Gadchiroli, India. *Indian Pediatrics*, 38:952-65.

Bang, A.T., R.A. Bang, M. Baitule et al. n.d. High prevalence and wide spectrum of reproductive morbidities in males in Gadchiroli, India, unpublished.

Bansal, R.K. 1992. Sexual behaviour and substance use patterns amongst adolescent truck cleaners and risk of HIV/AIDS. *Indian Journal of Maternal and Child Health,* 3(4): 108-10.

Bansal, R.K. 1995. Truck drivers and risk of STDs including HIV. *Indian Journal of Community Medicine*, 20: 28-30.

Barge, S. 2002. A multi-state abortion facility analysis: Experience from Maharashtra and Haryana. Paper presented at the Population Council workshop on 'Abortion in India: How Can Research Help Us Move Forward?' Goa.

Barge, S. and L. Ramachandar. 1999. Provider-client interactions in primary health care: A case study from Madhya Pradesh. In M.A. Koenig and M.E. Khan, eds., *Improving Quality of Care in India's Family Welfare Programme: The Challenge Ahead:* 92-116. New York: Population Council.

Barge, S., K. Manjunath and S. Nair. 1994. *Situation Analysis of MTP Facilities in Gujarat.* Vadodara: Centre for Operations Research and Training.

Barge, S., N. Kumar, G. Philips et al. 1997. *Situation Analysis of MTP Services in Uttar Pradesh.* Vadodara: Centre for Operations Research and Training.

Barge, S., M.E. Khan, S. Rajagopal et al. 1998. Availability and quality of MTP services in Gujarat, Maharashtra, Tamil Nadu and Uttar Pradesh: An in-depth study. Paper presented at the International Workshop on 'Abortion Facilities and Post-Abortion Care in the Context of the RCH Programme,' New Delhi.

Baru, R. 2003. Policy analysis of health sector reforms in India. Paper presented at the National Seminar on 'Global Agendas, Local

Realities: Implications of Health Sector Reforms on Woman's Access to Reproductive Health Services in India,' New Delhi, 7 March.

Barua, A. 2000. Reproductive health needs of married adolescent girls in rural Maharashtra. Paper presented at the Workshop on 'Reproductive Health in India: New Evidence and Issues,' Pune, 28 February-1 March.

Barua, A. 2002. Availability and accessibility of abortion care: Provider perspectives. Paper presented at the Population Council Workshop on 'Abortion in India: How Can Research Help Us Move Forward?' Goa.

Barua, A. and K. Kurz. 2001. Reproductive health-seeking by married adolescent girls in Maharashtra, India. *Reproductive Health Matters*, 9(17): 53-62.

Basu, D.P. 1994. Appropriate methodologies for studying sexual behaviour in India. *Indian Journal of Social Work*, 55(4): 573-88.

Baveja, R., K. Buckshee, K. Das et al. 2000. Evaluating contraceptive choice through the method-mix approach: An Indian Council of Medical Research Task Force study. *Contraception*, 61: 113-19.

Bhandari, N. and S. Mayank. 1999. A study on the perceptions, prevalence and health seeking behaviour of maternal morbidities in an urban slum. Unpublished report.

Bharat, S. 1999. *HIV/AIDS Related Discrimination, Stigmatisation and Denial in India: A Study in Mumbai and Bangalore*. Mumbai: Tata Institute of Social Sciences.

Bharat, S. and P. Aggleton. 1999. Facing the challenge: Household responses to HIV/AIDS in Mumbai, India. *AIDS Care*, 1: 31-44.

Bhathena, R.K., N.K. Sheriar and J. Guillebaud. 1990. Late abortion practice in teaching hospitals in India. *Journal of Obstetrics and Gynaecology*, 10(4): 299-303.

Bhatia, J.C. 1988. *A Study of Maternal Mortality in Anantpur District, Andhra Pradesh, India*. Bangalore: Indian Institute of Management.

Bhatia, J.C. 1993. Levels and causes of maternal mortality in Southern India. *Studies in Family Planning*, 24(5): 310-18.

Bhatia, J.C. 1995. Levels and determinants of maternal morbidity: Results from a community-based study in southern India. *International Journal of Gynaecology and Obstetrics*, 50, supplement 2: S153-63.

Bhatia, J.C. and J. Cleland. 1995. Self-reported symptoms of gynaecological morbidity and their treatment in south India. *Studies in Family Planning*, 26(4): 203-16.

Bhatia, J.C. and J. Cleland. 1996. Obstetric morbidity in South India: Results from a community survey. *Social Science and Medicine*, 43(10): 1507-16.

Bhatia, J.C. and J. Cleland. 2001. Health care seeking and expenditure by young Indian mothers in the public and private sectors. *Health Policy and Planning*, 16(1): 55-61.

Bhatia, J.C., J. Cleland, L. Bhagavan et al. 1997. Levels and determinants of gynaecological morbidity in a district of south India. *Studies in Family Planning*, 28(2): 95-103.

Bhatnagar, P., V. Kashyap, D.K. Das et al. 1991. Clinico-epidemiological study of condylomatous lesions in inflammatory smears. *Journal of Obstetrics and Gynaecology of India,* 41(6): 793-98

Bhende, A.A. 1994. A study of sexuality of adolescent girls and boys in underprivileged groups in Bombay. *Indian Journal of Social Work*, 55: 557-71.

Bhujwala, R.A., B. Mishra, N.C. Bhargava et al. 1984. Non-gonococcal urethritis in men and its response to therapy. *Indian Journal of Medical Research,* 79:728-32.

Bhujwala, R.A., T.D. Biswas, V. Bhargava et al. 1988. Detection of chlamydial and gonococcal antibodies in women with pelvic inflammatory disease and infertility: An aid to diagnosis. *Journal of Obstetrics and Gynaecology of India*, 38(1): 96-99.

Bloom, S.S., T. Lippeveld and D. Wypij. 1999. Does antenatal care make a difference to safe delivery? A study in urban Uttar Pradesh. *Health Policy and Planning*, 14(1): 38-48.

Bloom, S.S., A.O. Tsui, M. Plotkin et al. 2000. What husbands in Northern India know about reproductive health: Correlates of knowledge about pregnancy and maternal and sexual health. *Journal of Biosocial Science*, 32(2): 237-51.

Bloom, S.S., D. Wypij and M. Das Gupta. 2001. Dimensions of women's autonomy and the influence on maternal health care utilisation in a north Indian city. *Demography*, 38(1): 67-78.

Booth, B., M. Verma and R. Beri. 1994. Foetal sex determination in infants in Punjab, India: Correlation and implications. *British Medical Journal*, 309(6964): 1259-61.

Bose, A. 2003. Fighting HIV/AIDS: Current scenario based on HIV sentinel rounds. *Health for the Millions*, 28(6): 26-27.

Brabin L., A. Gogate, S. Gogate et al. 1998. Reproductive tract infections, gynaecological morbidity and HIV seroprevalence among women in Mumbai, India. *Bulletin of World Health Organisation,* 76: 277-87.

Brown, A., S.J. Jejeebhoy, I. Shah et al. 2001. Sexual relations among young people in developing countries: Evidence from WHO case studies. *Occasional Papers of the Department of Reproductive Health and Research, World Health Organisation, No 4 (WHO/RHR/01.8).*

Bryan, A.D., J.D. Fisher and T.J. Benziger. 2000. HIV prevention information, motivation, behavioural skills and behaviour among truck drivers in Chennai, India. *AIDS*, 14(6): 756-58.

Buch, N. 2003. Panchayati raj and the two-child norm: Implications and consequences. Preliminary findings. Mahila Chetna Manch, unpublished.

Bultreys, M. et al. 2002. Advances in the prevention of mother-to-child HIV transmission: Current issues, future challenges. *AIDScience*, 2(4).

Carolina Population Centre. 1997. *Uttar Pradesh Male Reproductive Health Survey 1995-1996*. Carolina Population Centre, North Carolina.

Cates, W., T.M.M. Farely and P.J. Rowe. 1985a. Worldwide patterns of infertility: Is Africa different? *Lancet*, 14 September: 596-98.

Cates W., T.M.M. Farely and P.J. Rowe. 1985b. Patterns of infertility in the developed and developing worlds. In P.J. Rowe and V.M. Ekaterina, eds., *Diagnosis and Treatment of Infertility*. Bern: Hans Huber Publishers.

Chakrabarti, V. 2003. Population education in formal and non-formal sectors in India. In S. Bott et al., eds., *Towards Adulthood: Exploring the Sexual and Reproductive Health of Adolescents in South Asia:* 165-67. Geneva: World Health Organisation.

Chakrabarti, S., S. Panda, A. Chatterjee et al. 2000. HIV-1 subtypes in injecting drug users and their non-injecting wives in Manipur, India. *Indian Journal of Medical Research*, 111:189-94.

Chandiramani, R. 1998. A view from the field: Phone helpline in India helps identify HIV risk behaviours. *SIECUS Report*, 26(5): 4-6.

Char, A. and S. Vaidya. 2000. Gynaecological morbidity among women seeking sterilization services in rural Maharashtra. Paper presented at the Workshop on 'Reproductive Health in India: New Evidence and Issues', Pune, 28 February-1 March.

Chatterjee, M. 1996. Addressing gender and poverty concerns in a reproductive health programme. In A.R. Measham and R.A. Heaver, eds., *Supplement to India's Family Welfare Programme: Moving to a Reproductive and Child Health Approach.* Washington, D.C.: World Bank.

Chaudhary, S.D., K.K. Bhattia, R.K. Bansal et al. 1988. Pattern of sexually transmitted diseases in Rohtak. *Indian Journal of Sexually Transmitted Disease,* 9: 4-7.

Chaudhuri, P. and R. Iyengar. 1994. *Chlamydia trachomatis* infection in a South Indian population: A prospective pilot study. *Journal of Obstetrics and Gynaecology of India*, 44(4): 593-94.

Chawla, M. 1996. *Dual Job-holding by Public Sector Physicians in India.* Boston: Harvard School of Public Health.

Chhabra, S. and L. Fali. 1992. Clinical genital infection in infertile women with *Chlamydia trachomatis* infection. *Journal of Obstetrics and Gynaecology of India*, 42(1): 68-70.

Chhabra, R. and S.C. Nuna. 1994. *Abortion in India: An Overview.* New Delhi: Veeremdra Printers.

Chhabra, S., N. Gupte, A. Mehta et al. 1988. MTP and concurrent contraceptive adoption in rural India. *Studies in Family Planning*, 19(4): 244-47.

Chhabra, S., G. Swarup, K. Swarup et al. 1991. Correlation of cervical abnormalities with abnormal smears in mass screening programme of cervical cytology. *Journal of Obstetrics and Gynaecology of India*, 41(5): 681-83.

Chhabra, S., K. Aher, P. Narang et al. 1993. *Chlamydia trachomatis* infection and cervical intraepithelial neoplasia. *Journal of Obstetrics and Gynaecology of India*, 43(1): 93-94.

Chopra, A., R.R. Mittal, P. Singh et al. 1990. Patterns of sexually transmitted diseases at Patiala. *Indian Journal of Sexually Transmitted Diseases,* 11: 43-45.

Collumbien, M., B. Das and O.M.R. Campbell. 2001. Why are condoms used, and how many are needed? Estimates from Orissa, India. *International Family Planning Perspectives*, 27(4): 171-77, 216.

Collumbien, M., B. Das, N. Bohidar et al. 2000. Male sexual behaviour in Orissa. Paper presented at the Workshop on 'Reproductive Health in India: New Evidence and Issues,' Pune, 28 February-1 March.

Coyaji, K. 2002. Medical Abortion. Paper presented at the Population Council Workshop on 'Abortion in India: How Can Research Help Us Move Forward?' Goa.

Coyaji, K., B. Elul, U. Krishna et al. 2001. Mifepristone abortion outside the urban research hospital setting in India [research letter]. *Lancet,* 357: 120-22.

Coyaji, K., B. Elul, U. Krishna et al. 2002. Mifepristone-misoprostol abortion: A trial in rural and urban Maharashtra, India. *Contraception,* 66: 33-40.

Daga, A.S., S.J. Jejeebhoy and S. Rajgopal. 1998. *Domestic Violence against Women: An Investigation of Hospital Casualty Records, Mumbai.* Paper presented at CEHAT International Conference on 'Preventing Violence, Caring for Survivors,' November.

Damayanthi, K. 2003. Presentation on sharing of AP experience on AIDS Prevention Education Programme (APEP). AP SACS, Hyderabad.

Das Gupta, M. 1987. Selective discrimination against female children in rural Punjab, India. *Population and Development Review,* 13(1).

Das Gupta, M., L.C. Chen and T.N. Krishnan. 1995. *Women's Health in India: Risk and Vulnerability*. Mumbai: Oxford University Press.

Datta, K.K., R.S. Sharma, P.M.A. Razack et al. 1980. Morbidity patterns amongst rural pregnant women in Alwar, Rajasthan: A cohort study. *Health and Population: Perspectives and Issues*, 3(4): 282-92.

Deb, M., T. Kaur, K. Prakash et al. 1989. Incidence of *Gardnerella vaginalis* in non-specific vaginitis, *Journal of Obstetrics and Gynaecology of India*, 39(1): 88-92.

Deepak Charitable Trust. 2000. *Male Semen Loss Concerns: A Report.* Vadodara: Deepak Charitable Trust.

Deorari, A.K., V.K. Paul, M. Singh et al. 2000. The national movement of neonatal resuscitation in India. *Journal of Tropical Pediatrics,* 46: 315-17.

Desai, P., V. Shrinivasan and M. Hazra. 1992. Understanding the emotions of infertile couples. *Journal of Obstetrics and Gynaecology of India,* 42: 498-503.

Desai, V.K., J.K. Kosambiya, H.G. Thakor et al. 2003. Prevalence of sexually transmitted infections and performance of STI syndromes against aetiological diagnosis in female sex workers of red light area in Surat, India. *Sexually Transmitted Infections*, 79(2): 111-15.

DFID/FHI. 2001a. *Prevalence of Sexually Transmitted Infections and HIV among Long Distance Inter-city Truck Drivers and Helpers of Southern India.* New Delhi: FHI.

DFID/FHI. 2001b. *Prevalence of Sexually Transmitted Infections and HIV among Long Distance Inter-city Truck Drivers and Helpers of Eastern India.* New Delhi: FHI.

DFID/FHI 2001c. *Prevalence of Sexually Transmitted Infections and HIV among Long Distance Inter-city Truck Drivers and Helpers of Northern India.* New Delhi: FHI.

DFID/FHI. 2001d. *Behavioural Surveillance Survey in Healthy Highway Project, India: Summary Report.* New Delhi: FHI.

DFID/FHI. 2001e. *Health Care Provider Survey in Healthy Highway Project, India: Summary Report.* New Delhi: FHI.

DFID/KSACS/FHI. 2001a. *Prevalence of Sexually Transmitted Infections and HIV among Female Sex Workers of Calicut, Kerala, India.* New Delhi: FHI.

DFID/GSACS/FHI. 2001b. *Prevalence of Sexually Transmitted Infections and HIV among Female Sex Workers of Ahmedabad, Gujarat, India.* New Delhi: FHI.

DFID/GSACS/FHI. 2001c. *Prevalence of Sexually Transmitted Infections and HIV among Female Sex Workers of Surat, Gujarat, India.* New Delhi: FHI.

DFID/KSACS/FHI. 2001d. *Prevalence of Sexually Transmitted Infections and HIV among Female Sex Workers of Trivandrum, Kerala, India.* New Delhi: FHI.

DFID/KSACS/FHI. 2001e. *Prevalence of Sexually Transmitted Infections and HIV among Female Sex Workers of Trissur, Kerala, India.* New Delhi: FHI.

DFID/APSACS/FHI 2001f. *Prevalence of Sexually Transmitted Infections and HIV among Female Sex Workers of Kakinad and Peddapuram, Andhra Pradesh, India.* New Delhi: FHI.

DFID/APSACS/FHI. 2001g. *Health Care Provider Survey in Andhra Pradesh, India: Summary Report.* New Delhi: FHI.

DFID/GSACS/FHI. 2001h. *Health Care Provider Survey in Gujarat, India: Summary Report.* New Delhi: FHI.

DFID/KSACS/FHI. 2001i. *Health Care Provider Survey in Kerala, India: Summary Report.* New Delhi: FHI.

DFID/IIAPCP/FHI/AVERT. 2001j. *Health Care Provider Survey in Maharashtra.* New Delhi: FHI.

DFID/OSACS/FHI. 2001k. *Health Care Provider Survey in Orissa, India: Summary Report.* New Delhi: FHI.

Dhall, K., A. Sarkar, C. Sokhey et al. 1990. Incidence of gonococcal infection and its clinicopathological correlation in patients attending gynaecological out-patient department. *Journal of Obstetrics and Gynaecology of India*, 40(3): 410-13.

Dharmalingam, A. 1995. The social context of family planning in a south Indian village. *International Family Planning Perspectives*, 21(3): 98-103.

Divekar, A.A., A.S. Gogate, L.K. Shivkar et al. 2000. Disease prevalence in women attending the STD clinic in Mumbai (formerly Bombay), India. *International Journal of STD and AIDS*, 11: 45-48.

Duraisamy, P., C.C. Daly, R.K. Homan et al. 2003. Economic impact of HIV/AIDS on patients and households in South India: Costs and burden on households and coping strategies. Paper presented at 'IAEN Annual Conference, Current Issues in the Economics of HIV/AIDS,' Washington, D.C., 24-25 April.

Durbar Mahila Samanwaya Committee (DMSC). 1998. *The Fallen Learn to Rise: The Social Impact of STD/HIV Intervention Programme*. Calcutta.

Duvvury, N., M. Nayak and K. Allendorf. 2002. Links between masculinity and violence: Aggregate analysis. In *Domestic Violence in India 4: Exploring Strategies, Promoting Dialogue. Men Masculinities and Domestic Violence in India: Summary Report of Four Studies*. Washington, D.C.: International Centre for Research on Women.

Eicher, A.D., N. Crofts, S. Benjamin et al. 2000. A certain fate: Spread of HIV among young injecting drug users in Manipur, north-east India. *AIDS Care*, 12(4): 497-504.

Elul B., C. Ellertson and B. Winikoff. 1999. Side effects of mifepristone-misoprostol abortion versus surgical abortion: Data from a trial in China, Cuba and India. *Contraception*, 59: 107-14.

Elul B., S. Barge, S. Verma et al. 2003 (forthcoming). *Unintended Pregnancy and Abortion: A Community-based Study in Rajasthan-Summary Report*. New Delhi: Population Council.

EVALUATION Project. 1997. *Uttar Pradesh Male Reproductive Health Survey, 1995-96*. Chapel Hill: Carolina Population Centre, University of North Carolina.

Evans, C. and H. Lambert. 1997. Health seeking strategies and sexual health among female sex workers in urban India: Implications for research and service provision. *Social Science and Medicine*, 44(1): 1791-1803.

Farley, T.M.M. and E.M. Belsey. 1988. The prevalence and aetiology of infertility. Paper presented at the African Population Conference, sponsored by the IUSSP and the Central Statistical Office, Dakar, November.

Foo, G. and M. Koenig. 2000. Quality of care within the Indian family welfare programme. In R. Ramasubban and S.J. Jejeebhoy, eds., *Women's Reproductive Health in India*: 383-417. Jaipur: Rawat Publications.

Ganapathy, S., J. Ramakrishna and Z. Matthews. 2000. Birth rites and rituals: Intrapartum care and care seeking in rural Karnataka. In C. Puri and P.F.A. Van Look, eds., *Sexual and Reproductive Health: Recent Advances, Future Directions,* vol. 1: 309-25. New Delhi: New Age International.

Ganatra, B. 2000. Abortion research in India: What we know, and what we need to know. In R. Ramasubban and S.J. Jejeebhoy, eds., *Women's Reproductive Health in India:* 186-235. Jaipur: Rawat Publications.

Ganatra, B.R. and S.S. Hirve. 1995. Unsafe motherhood: The determinants of maternal mortality. *Journal of the Indian Medical Association*, 93(2): 34-35.

Ganatra, B.R. and S. Hirve. 2002a. Adolescents and induced abortion: Evidence from rural Maharashtra. Paper presented at the Population Council Workshop on 'Abortion in India: How Can Research Help Us Move Forward?' Goa.

Ganatra, B. and S. Hirve 2002b. Induced abortions among adolescent women in rural Maharashtra. *Reproductive Health Matters*, 10(19): 76-85.

Ganatra, B.R., K.J. Coyaji and V.N. Rao. 1996. *A Community-cum-hospital-based Case Control Study on Maternal Mortality: Final Report*. Pune: KEM Hospital Research Centre.

Ganatra, B.R., K.J. Coyaji and V.N. Rao. 1998. Too far, too little, too late: A community-based case control study of maternal mortality in rural West Maharashtra. *Bulletin of the World Health Organisation,* 76(6): 591-98.

Ganatra, B.R., S.S. Hirve and V.N. Rao. 2000. Sex-selective abortions: Evidence from a community-based study in western India. *Asia Pacific Population Journal*, 16(2): 109-24.

Gandotra, M.M. and N.P. Das. 1996. Factors influencing choice of a contraceptive and the reasons for its discontinuation. In M.E. Khan and G. Cernada, eds., *Spacing as an Alternative Strategy: India's Family Welfare Programme:* 95-114. New Delhi: B.R. Publishing Corporation.

Gangakhedkar, R.R., M.E. Bentley, A.D. Divekar et al. 1997. Spread of HIV infection in married monogamous women in India. *Journal of the American Medical Association*, 278(23): 2090-92.

Ganguli, D.D., V. Ramesh, S.A. Zaheer et al. 1985. Profile of gonorrhoea in males. *Indian Journal of Sexually Transmitted Diseases*, 6: 44-46.

Garg, S., N. Sharma, P. Bhalla et al. 2002. Reproductive morbidity in an Indian urban slum: Need for health action. *Sexually Transmitted Infections*, 78(1): 68-69.

Gawande, A.V., N.D. Vasudeo, S.P. Zodpey et al. 2000. Sexually transmitted infections in long distance truck drivers. *Journal of Communicable Diseases*, 32(3): 212-15.

George, A. and S. Jaswal. 1995. *Understanding Sexuality: Ethnographic Study of Poor Women in Bombay*. Women and AIDS Program Research Report Series No.12. Washington, D.C.: International Centre for Research on Women.

George, S. and R. Dhaiya. 1998. Female foeticide in rural Haryana. *Economic and Political Weekly*, 33(32): 2191-97.

George, S., M. Jacob, T.J. John et al. 1997. A case-control analysis of risk factors in HIV transmission in South India. *Journal of Acquired Immune Deficiency Syndromes and Human Retrovirology,* 14: 290-93.

Ghosh, M.D. 2003. HIV/AIDS in South Asia: Can we collaborate? *Health for the Millions,* 28(6): 4-9.

Ghosh, R. 2001. Intention not to use contraception: A comparative study of northern and southern states of India. *Demography India*, 30(2): 261-80.

Ghosh, M. and N.K. Das. 1990. Anonder Opekshay: Chondalika Ekdal Khokkosh (in Bengali), Calcutta Development Dialogue, Calcutta. Cited in M. Nag (1996), *Sexual Behaviour and AIDS in India*. New Delhi: Vikas Publishing House.

Giri, T.K., J.P. Wali, H.S. Meena et al. 1995. Socio-demographic characteristics of HIV infection in northern India. *Journal of Communicable Diseases*, 27(1): 1-9.

Gittelsohn, J., M.E. Bentley, P.J. Pelto et al. 1994. *Listening to Women Talk About Their Health: Issues and Evidence from India.* New Delhi: Har-Anand Publications.

Godinho, D., F. Dias-Saxena, G. Divan et al. 2002. *Sangath Biennial Report, 2000-2002*. Porvorim, Goa, Sangath Society for Child Development and Family Guidance.

Gogate, A., L. Brabin, S. Nicholas et al. 1998. Risk factors for laparoscopically confirmed pelvic inflammatory disease: Findings from Mumbai (Bombay). India. *Sexually Transmitted Infections*, 74: 426-32.

Gogate, A., L. Deodhar, R. Bhatt et al. 1990. Mycoplasma hominis infections in female genital tract and use of immunofluorescence for antibody detection. *Indian Journal of Medical Research,* 91(A): 364-67.

Gopalakrishnan, K., N. Prata, D. Montagu et al. 2002. NGOs providing low cost, high quality family planning and reproductive health service: Case study Janani. India. *Bay Area International Group Monograph Series,* 1:3-4.

Goparaju, L. 1993. Unplanned, unsafe: Male students' sexual behaviour. Paper presented at the workshop on 'Sexual Aspects of AIDS/STD Prevention in India,' Mumbai, 23-27 November.

Government of India (GOI). 2002. The Medical Termination of Pregnancy (Amendment) Bill (Bill No. XXXV).

Government of India (GOI). 2003. The Pre-Natal Diagnostic Techniques (Regulation And Prevention Of Misuse) Amendment Act (Act. No. 14).

Government of India (GOI), Department of Family Welfare and European Commission. 2001. Health and family welfare sector programme in India: Providing emergency obstetric care in India (final draft). *ECTA Working Paper,* 2001/48.

Government of Madhya Pradesh. 2000. *Madhya Pradesh Population Policy.* Department of Health and Family Welfare, Government of Madhya Pradesh.

Griffiths, P. and R. Stephenson. 2001. Understanding users' perspectives of barriers to maternal health care use in Maharashtra, India. *Journal of Biosocial Science,* 33(3): 339-59.

Gupta, J. 1993. People like you never agree to get it: An Indian family planning clinic. *Reproductive Health Matters,* 1: 39-43.

Gupta, J. 2000. *New Reproductive Technologies, Women's Health and Autonomy: Freedom or Dependency?* New Delhi: Sage Publications.

Gupta, I. and A. Mitra. 1999. Knowledge of HIV/AIDS among migrants in Delhi slums. *Journal of Health and Population in Developing Countries,* 2(1): 26-32.

Gupta, S.D. and P.M. Keyl. 1998. Effectiveness of prenatal tetanus-toxoid immunization against neonatal tetanus in a rural area in India. *Pediatric Infectious Disease Journal,* 17(4): 316-21.

Gupta, A.N., G.I. Dhall and L.K. Dhaliwal. 1983. Epidemiology of infertility in Chandigarh. In S. Shah Ratnam, Eng Soon Teoh and C. Anand Kumar, eds., *Advances in Infertility and Sterility,* vol. 4: 103-9. Singapore: Parthenon Publishing.

Gupta, V.M., R. Jain and P. Sen. 2001. Study of interspouse communication and adoption of family planning and immunization services in a rural block of Varanasi district. *Indian Journal of Public Health*, 45(4): 110-15.

Gupta, M.K., W.P. Thergaonkar and N. Chawla. 1998. Anonymous testing of HIV infection in pregnant women. *Journal of Communicable Diseases*, 30(2): 121-22.

Gupte, M., S. Bandewar and H. Pisal. 1996. Women's role in decision making in abortion: Profiles from rural Maharashtra. Unpublished paper. Centre for Enquiry Into Health and Allied Themes (CEHAT).

Gupte, M., S. Bandewar and H. Pisal. 1997. Abortion needs of women in India: A case study of rural Maharashtra. *Reproductive Health Matters*, 9 (May): 77-86.

Gupte, M., S. Bandewar and H. Pisal. 1999. Women's perspective on the quality of care: Evidence from rural Maharashtra. In M.A. Koenig and M.E. Khan, eds., *Quality of Care Within the Indian Family Welfare Programme:*117-39. New York: Population Council.

Haberland, N., E. McGrory and K.G. Santhya. 2001. First time parents project, Supplemental diagnostic report, Vadodara, unpublished.

Hawkes, S. and K.G. Santhya. 2001. Diverse realities: Understanding sexually transmitted infections and HIV in India. *Population Council Working PaperNo. 15*. New Delhi.

Hindustan Times. 2003. Abortion gets a medical edge. Sutirtho Partranobis, 13 March.

Hira, S.K. 1991. *Guidelines for Prevention of Adverse Outcomes of Pregnancy due to Syphilis*. Geneva: World Health Organisation.

Hirve, S.S. and B.R. Ganatra. 1994. Determinants of low birth weight: A community-based prospective cohort study. *Indian Paediatrics*, 31(10): 1221-25.

Hutton, I. 1996. Reduction of food intake during pregnancy in rural South India. *Tropical Medicine and International Health*, 1(3): 399-405.

India Today. 2003. Foetal extraction. Supriya Bezbaruah, 12 May.

Indian Council of Medical Research (ICMR). 1989. *Illegal Abortion in Rural Areas: A Task Force Study*. New Delhi: ICMR.

Indian Council of Medical Research (ICMR). 1991. *Evaluation of Quality of Family Welfare Services at Primary Health Centre Level: An ICMR Task force Study*. New Delhi: ICMR.

Indian Council of Medical Research (ICMR). 1997. A baseline survey of reproductive health services in 23 districts (14 states) of India. New Delhi: ICMR.

Indian Council of Medical Research (ICMR). 2000. Need and feasibility of providing assisted technologies for infertility management in resource-poor settings. *ICMR Bulletin*, 3: 6-7.

Indian Council of Medical Research and National Academy of Medical Sciences (ICMR and NAMS). 2002. National Guidelines for Accreditation, Supervision and Regulation of ART Clinics in India. Draft Report, New Delhi.

Indian Council of Medical Research Task Force on IUD and Hormonal Contraceptives. 1994. Improved utilization of spacing methods-intrauterine devices (IUDs) and low-dose combined oral contraceptives (OCs)-through reorientation training for improving quality of services. *Contraception*, 50: 215-28.

Indian Institute for Health Management and Research (IIHMR). 2000. *Financing Reproductive and Child Health Care in Rajasthan*. New Delhi: USAID.

International Clinical Epidemiologists Network (INCLEN). 2000. *Domestic Violence in India 3: A Summary Report of a Multi-Site Household Survey*. Washington, D.C.: International Centre for Research on Women and Centre for Development and Population Activities.

International Institute for Population Sciences (IIPS). 1995. *National Family Health Survey (MCH and Family Planning), India, 1992-93*. Mumbai: IIPS.

International Institute for Population Sciences (IIPS). 2001a. *Reproductive and Child Health Project: Rapid Household Survey (Phase I and II), 1998-99*. Mumbai: IIPS.

International Institute for Population Sciences (IIPS). 2001b. *India Facility Survey (Under Reproductive and Child Health Project) Phase I 1999*, Mumbai: IIPS.

International Institute for Population Sciences (IIPS) and ORC Macro. 2000. *National Family Health Survey (NFHS-2), 1998-99; India*. Mumbai: IIPS.

International Labour Organisation (ILO). 1998. *Yearbook of Labour Statistics 1998*. Geneva: International Labour Organisation.

Iyengar, K. and S. Iyengar. 1999. Dealing with infertility: Experience of a reproductive health programme in southern Rajasthan. Paper presented at the UNFPA Consultation on 'Infertility Prevention and Management,' New Delhi.

Iyengar K. and S. Iyengar. 2002. Experience with manual vacuum aspiration in a rural primary health care setting. Paper presented at the Population Council Workshop on 'Abortion in India: How Can Research Help Us Move Forward?' Goa.

Jacob, M. 1992. STDs among HIV patients of a referral hospital in India and their role in the transmission of HIV. Paper presented at the Eighth International Conference on 'AIDS/Third STD World Congress,'Amsterdam, 17-25 July.

Jacob, M., P.S.S. Rao, G. Sridharan et al. 1989. Epidemiology and clinical profile of genital herpes. *Indian Journal of Medical Research*, 89: 4-11.

Jain, A.K. 1989. Fertility reduction and the quality of family planning services. *Studies in Family Planning*, 20(1): 1-16.

Jana, S. 1992. No title. Abstract published for the 2nd International Congress on AIDS in Asia and the Pacific, Randwick, Australia, AIDS Society of Asia and the Pacific, p. 105. Cited in M. Nag (1996), *Sexual Behaviour and AIDS in India*. New Delhi: Vikas Publishing House.

Jana, S. 1995. Three years' stint at Sonagachi: An exposition. Paper distributed at the Indo-US Workshop on 'Behavioural Research Priorities: Developing Effective Strategies for the Prevention of HIV in India,' Tata Institute of Social Sciences, Mumbai, 24-29 April. Cited in M. Nag (1996), *Sexual Behaviour and AIDS in India*. New Delhi: Vikas Publishing House.

Jana, S., N. Bandyopadhyay, S. Mukherjee et al. 1998. STD/HIV intervention with sex workers in West Bengal, India. *AIDS*, 12(suppl B): S101-S108.

Jaswal, S. 2000. Health records and domestic violence in Thane district, Maharashtra. *Domestic Violence in India 2: A Summary report of Four Records Studies.* Washington, D.C.: International Centre for Research on Women and Centre for Development and Population Activities.

Jayarao, P., A. Gogate, L. Deodhar et al. 1989. Trichomoniasis: A clinical and laboratory evaluation. *Journal of Obstetrics and Gynaecology of India*, 39(6): 829-33.

Jeffery, P., R. Jeffery and A. Lyon. 1989. *Labour Pains and Labour Power: Women and Childbearing in India.* London: Zed Books.

Jejeebhoy, S.J. 1990. Measuring contraceptive use-failure and continuation: An overview of new approaches. In *Measuring the Dynamics of*

Contraceptive Use: Proceedings of the United Nations Expert Group Meeting: 21-45. New York: United Nations.

Jejeebhoy, S.J. 1996. *Adolescent Sexual and Reproductive Behaviour: A Review of the Evidence from India.* Washington, D.C.: International Centre for Research on Women.

Jejeebhoy, S.J. 1998a. Associations between wife-beating and fetal and infant death: Impressions from a survey in rural India. *Studies in Family Planning,* 29(3): 300-8.

Jejeebhoy, S.J. 1998b. Wife beating in rural India: A husband's right? Evidence from survey data. *Economical and Political Weekly,* 33 (15): 855-62.

Jejeebhoy, S.J. 2000a. Adolescent sexual and reproductive behaviour: A review of the evidence from India. In R. Ramasubban and S. Jejeebhoy, eds., *Women's Reproductive Health in India*: 40-101. Jaipur: Rawat Publications.

Jejeebhoy, S.J. 2000b. Women's autonomy in rural India: Its dimensions, determinants and the influence of context. In H. Presser and G. Sen, eds., *Female Empowerment and Demographic Processes: Moving Beyond Cairo.* Oxford: Clarendon Press.

Jejeebhoy, S.J. 2000c. Empower women, ensure choices: Key to enhancing reproductive health. In C. Puri and P.F.A. Van Look, eds., *Sexual and Reproductive Health: Recent Advances, Future Directions,* vol. 1: 177-217. New Delhi: New Age International.

Jejeebhoy, S.J. and M. Sebastian. 2003. Actions that protect: Promoting sexual and reproductive health and choice among young people in India. *Population Council South and East Asia Regional Working Paper No. 18,* New Delhi.

Jejeebhoy, S.J. and M.A. Koenig. 2003. The social context of gynaecological morbidity: Correlates, consequences and health seeking behaviour. In S.J. Jejeebhoy, M.A. Koenig and C. Elias, eds., *Reproductive Tract Infections and Other Gynaecological Disorders: A Multidisciplinary Research Approach*: 30-81. Cambridge: Cambridge University Press.

Jejeebhoy, S.J. and S. Kulkarni. 1996. Promoting contraceptive choices in the Indian programme: Women's perspectives. In M.E. Khan and G. Cernada, eds., *Spacing as an Alternative Strategy: India's Family Welfare Programme*: 31-52. New Delhi: B.R. Publishing Corporation.

Jesani, A. 2001. Baseline information on trend and result indicators for maternal mortality and morbidity. Report to the MacArthur Foundation.

Jindal, U.N. and G.I. Dhall. 1990. Psychosexual problems of infertile women in India. *International Journal of Fertility*, 35: 222-25.

Jindal, U.N. and A.N. Gupta. 1989. Social problems of infertile women in India. *International Journal of Fertility*, 34: 30-33.

John, T.J., P.G. Babu, N.K. Saraswati et al. 1993. The epidemiology of AIDS in the Vellore region, southern India. *AIDS*, 7(3): 421-24.

Johnston, H.B. 2002. *Abortion Practice in India: A Review of the Literature*. Mumbai: CEHAT.

Joseph, A., J. Prasad and S. Abraham. 2003. Gynaecological problems among young married women in Tamil Nadu, India. In S. Bott et al., eds., *Towards Adulthood: Exploring the Sexual and Reproductive Health of Adolescents in South Asia*: 138-41. Geneva: World Health Organisation.

Joseph, A., R.A. Srikanth, S. Abraham et al. 1998. Sexual behavior: Older husbands, younger wives. Paper presented at the workshop on 'Men as Supportive Partners in Reproductive and Sexual Health,' Kathmandu, 23-26 June.

Joseph, G.A., S. Bhattacharji, A. Joseph et al. 1997. General and reproductive health of adolescent girls in rural South India. *Indian Pediatrics*, 34(3): 242-45.

Joshi, P.L. 2003. National response to HIV/AIDS epidemic in India. *Health for the Millions*, 28(6): 10-13.

Joshi, J.V., S. Palayekar, K.T. Hazari et al. 1994. The prevalence of *Chlamydia trachomatis* in young women. *National Medical Journal of India*, 7(2): 57-59.

Kakar, D.N. 1983. Traditional healers in North India: A case study. *Nursing Journal of India*, 74: 61-63.

Kamat, H.A. and D.D. Banker. 1993. Human immunodeficiency virus-1 infection among patients with sexually transmitted diseases in Bombay. *National Medical Journal of India*, 6(1): 11-13.

Kanani, S., K. Latha and M. Shah. 1994. Application of qualitative methodologies to investigate perceptions of women and health practitioners regarding women's health disorders in Baroda slums. In J. Gittelsohn et al., eds., *Listening to Women Talk about their Health: Issues and Evidence from India*: 116-30. New Delhi: Har-Anand Publications.

Kantharaj, K., T.E. Mertens, G.D. Smith et al. 1995. Sexually transmitted disease services in Madras: Could their role in AIDS prevention be strengthened? *Indian Journal of Public Health*, 29(3): 93-98.

Kapoor, S.K., V.P. Reddaiah and J. Lobo. 1985. Antenatal care and perinatal mortality. *Indian Journal of Paediatrics*, 52 (415): 159-62.

Kapoor, R.K., A.K. Srivastava, P.K. Misra et al. 1996. Perinatal mortality in urban slums in Lucknow. *Indian Paediatrics,* 33(1): 19-23.

Kar, J., P.L. Agarwal, S.D. Mishra et al. 1988. Vaginal cytology in erosion of cervix and cervicitis, *Journal of Obstetrics and Gynaecology of India*, 38(1): 100-5.

Kaur, U., S.P. Sahni, P. Bembery et al. 1996. Sexual behaviour, drug use and Hepatitis B infection in Chandigarh students, *National Medical Journal of India,* 9(4): 156-59.

Kerrigan, M., L. Gaffikin and R. Magarick. 1995. *Post-Abortion Care Services in Uttar Pradesh State, India*. Baltimore: Johns Hopkins.

Khan, S. 1994. Cultural contexts of sexual behaviour and identities and their impact upon preventive models: An overview of South Asian men who have sex with men. *Indian Journal of Social Work*, 55(4): 633-46.

Khan, M.E. and B. C. Patel. 1997. *Male Involvement in Family Planning: A Knowledge Attitude Behaviour and Practice Survey of Agra District.* New Delhi: Population Council.

Khan, M.E., S. Barge and G. Philip. 1996. Abortion in India: An overview. *Social Change*, 26(3-4): 208-25.

Khan, M.E., I. Khan and N. Mukerjee. 1997. Involving men in safe motherhood. *Journal of Family Welfare*, 43(2): 18-30.

Khan, M.E., B.C. Patel and R. Chandrasekhar. 1993. Abortion acceptors in India: Observations from a prospective study. In *Proceedings of the International Population Conference*: 253-68. IUSSP, vol. 1, Montreal.

Khan, M.E., R.B. Gupta and B.C. Patel. 1999. The quality and coverage of family planning services in Uttar Pradesh: Client perspectives. In M.A. Koenig and M.E. Khan, eds., *Improving Quality of Care in India's Family Welfare Programme: The Challenge Ahead*: 49-69. New York: Population Council.

Khan, M.E., B. C. Patel and R. B. Gupta. 1999. The quality of family planning services in Uttar Pradesh from the perspectives of service providers. In M.A. Koenig and M.E. Khan, eds., *Improving Quality of Care in India's Family Welfare Programme: The Challenge Ahead*: 238-72. New York: Population Council.

Khan, M.E., R. Anker, S.K. Ghosh et al. 1988. Inequalities between men and women in nutrition and family welfare services: An in-depth enquiry in an Indian village. *Social Action,* 38:

Khan, M.E., J.W. Townsend, R. Sinha et al. 1997. Sexual violence within marriage: A case study of rural Uttar Pradesh. Presented at the Annual Meeting of the American Public Health Association, Indianapolis.

Khan, M.E., S. Rajagopal, S. Barge et al. 1998. Situation analysis of MTP services in Gujarat, Maharashtra, Tamil Nadu and Uttar Pradesh. Paper presented at the International Workshop on 'Abortion Facilities and Post-abortion Care and Operation Research,' New York, 19-21 January.

Khan, M.E., S. Barge, N. Kumar et al. 1999. Abortion in India: Current situation and future challenges. In S. Pachauri, ed., *Implementing a Reproductive Health Agenda in India: The Beginning*: 507-29. New Delhi: Population Council.

Khandait, D.W., N.N. Ambadakar, S.P. Zodpey et al. 2000. Maternal age as a risk factor for stillbirth. *Indian Journal of Public Health*, 44(1): 28-30.

Khanna, S. 1997. Traditions and reproductive technology in an urbanizing north Indian village. *Social Science and Medicine,* 44(2): 171-80.

Kochar, M. 1980. Etiology of pelvic infections treated by the gynecologic service of the Kasturba Hospital, Delhi, India. *American Journal of Obstetrics and Gynecology,* 138(7) Pt 2: 872-74.

Koenig, M., S. Jejeebhoy, S. Singh et al. 1998. Investigating gynaecological morbidity in India: Not just another KAP survey. *Reproductive Health Matters,* 6(11): 84-97.

Kotecha, P.V., R.K. Baxi, S. Shah et al. 1999. Health-seeking behaviour of patients with pelvic inflammatory disease visiting a tertiary hospital at Vadodara (unpublished).

Krishna, U.R. 1995. The status of women and safe motherhood. *Journal of the Indian Medical Association*, 93(2): 34-35.

Kulkarni, S. 2003. The reproductive health status of married adolescents as assessed by NFHS-2, India. In S. Bott et al., eds., *Towards Adulthood: Exploring the Sexual and Reproductive Health of Adolescents in South Asia:* 55-58. Geneva: World Health Organisation.

Kulkarni, V., S. Kulkarni, N. Sahasrabudhe et al. 2000. Networks, language and sexual behaviours of men who have sex with men in an urban setting. Paper presented at the workshop on 'Reproductive Health in India: New Evidence and Issues,' Pune, 28 February-1 March.

Kumar, V., B.R. Garg and M.C. Baruah. 1990. A clinical study of genital ulcers. *Indian Journal of Sexually Transmitted Diseases*, 11:15-18.

Kumar, R.M., D.E. Rizk and A.K. Khurranna. 1997. AIDS in pregnancy among Indian tribal women. *International Journal of Gynaecology and Obstetrics*, 56(1): 59-60.

Kumar, R., M.M. Singh and M. Kaur. 1997. Impact of health centre availability on utilisation of maternity care and pregnancy outcome in a rural area of Haryana. *Journal of the Indian Medical Association*, 95(8): 448-50.

Kumar, R.M., S.A. Uduman and A.K. Khurranna. 1995. Impact of maternal HIV-1 infection on perinatal outcome. *International Journal of Gynaecology and Obstetrics*, 49(2): 137-43.

Kumar, A., M. Mehra, S.K. Badhan et al. 1997. Heterosexual behaviour and condom usage in an urban population of Delhi, India. *AIDS Care*, 9(3): 311-18.

Kumar, M.S., S. Mudaliar, S.P. Thyagarajan et al. 2000a. Rapid assessment and response to injecting drug use in Madras, South India. *International Journal of Drug Policy,* 11(1-2): 83-98.

Kumar, R., A. Raizada, A.K. Aggarwal et al. 2000b. Adolescent behaviour regarding reproductive health. *Indian Journal of Pediatrics*, 67(12): 877-81.

Kumar, B., B. Sahoo, S. Gupta et al. 2002. Rising incidence of genital herpes over two decades in a sexually transmitted disease clinic in north India. *Journal of Dermatology*, 29(2): 74-78.

Kunte, A., V. Misra, R. Paranjape et al. 1999. HIV seroprevalence and awareness about AIDS among pregnant women in rural areas of Pune district, Maharashtra, India. *Indian Journal of Medical Research*, 110:115-22.

Kura, M.M., S. Hira, M. Kohli et al. 1998. High occurrence of HBV among STD clinic attenders in Bombay, India. *International Journal of STD and AIDS*, 9: 231-33.

Kushtagi, P., K. Rao, E. Abraham et al. 1991. Prevalence of antibodies to chlamydia trachomatis among infertile couples. *Journal of Obstetrics and Gynaecology of India*, 41: 671-73.

Kusiako, T., C. Ronsmans and L. Van der Paal. 2000. Perinatal mortality attributable to complications of childbirth in Matlab, Bangladesh. *Bulletin of the World Health Organisation*, 78: 621-27.

Lawyer's Collective. 2002. *Campaign for a Civil Law on Domestic Violence.* New Delhi: Lawyer's Collective, Women's Rights Initiative.

Leslie, J. 1991. Women's nutrition: The key to improving health in developing countries? *Health Policy and Planning,* 6(1): 1-19.

Levine, R.E., H.E. Cross, S. Chhabra et al. 1992. Quality of health and family planning services in rural Uttar Pradesh: The clients' view. *Demography India,* 21(2): 247-66.

Levitt-Dayal, M. 2002. Role of NGOs in RCH services: Policy and partnership implications. In *Workshop Proceedings: Reproductive and Child Health and Population Policy Issues in Uttaranchal*, 2-3 May. Dehradun, Department of Health and Family Welfare, Government of Uttaranchal and Policy Project, Futures Group International.

Levitt-Dayal, M., R. Motihar, S. Kanani et al. 2003. Adolescent girls in India choose a better future: An impact assessment of an educational programme.In S. Bott et al., eds., *Towards Adulthood: Exploring the Sexual and Reproductive Health of Adolescents in South Asia:* 187-89. Geneva: World Health Organisation.

Maitra, N. 1998. Unsafe abortion: Practices and solutions. Paper presented at the International Workshop on 'Abortion Facilities and Post-abortion Care in the Context of the RCH Programme,' New Delhi.

Malathi, J., H.N. Madhavan, K.L. Therese et al. 2002. Prevalence of *Chlamydia trachomatis* and *herpes simplex* virus in males with urethritis and females with cervicitis attending STD clinics. *Indian Journal of Medical Research*, 116: 58-63.

Malhotra, M., J.B. Sharma, S. Batra et al. 2002. Maternal and perinatal outcome in varying degrees of anaemia. *International Journal of Gynaecology and Obstetrics*, 79(2): 93-100.

Malhotra, A., S. Parasuraman, L. Nyblade et al. 2003. *Realizing Reproductive Choices and Rights: Abortion and Contraception in India.* International Centre for Research on Women (ICRW).

Mali, JJ-B., K. Hazari, S. Chitlange et al. 1991. Abnormal cytology indicating sexually transmitted diseases in women attending family welfare clinics. *Journal of Obstetrics and Gynaecology of India*, 41(4): 521-24.

Mallik, R. 2002. *India-Recent Developments Affecting Women's Reproductive Rights.* Centre for Health and Gender Equity (CHANGE).

Mallik, R. 2003. Introduction of emergency contraceptive pills in India: Beyond the magic bullet. Centre for Health and Gender Equity. Available online at: www.genderhealth.org.

Mane, P. and S.A. Maitra. 1992. AIDS prevention: The socio-cultural context in India, Bombay. Mumbai: Tata Institute of Social Sciences.

Mania-Pramanik, J., P.K. Meherji, J.S. Gokral et al. 2001. *Chlamydia trachomatis* infection in an urban setting. *Sexually Transmitted Infections*, 77: 141.

Manjunath, J.V., D.M. Thappa and T.J. Jaisankar. 2002. Sexually transmitted diseases and sexual lifestyles of long-distance truck drivers: A clinico-epidemiologic study in south India. *International Journal of STD and AIDS*, 13(9): 612-17.

Marfatia, Y.S., S. Barge, S. Parmar et al. 2000. Treatment seeking behaviours of STD cases attending skin and VD department and private clinics in Vadodara, unpublished.

Mari Bhat, P.N. 2002. Maternal mortality in India: An update. *Studies in Family Planning*, 33(3): 227-36.

Mari Bhat, P.N. and J. B. Hasalkar. 1996. Factors influencing IUD retention in northern Karnataká. In M.E. Khan and G. Cernada, eds., *Spacing as an Alternative Strategy: India's Family Welfare Programme:* 63-94. New Delhi: B.R. Publishing Corporation.

Mari Bhat, P.N., K. Navaneetham and S. Irudaya Rajan. 1995. Maternal mortality in India: Estimates from a regression model. *Studies in Family Planning*, 26(4): 217-32.

Martin, S., B. Kilgallen, A. Tsui et al. 1999. Sexual behaviours and reproductive health outcomes. *Journal of the American Medical Association*, 282(20): 1967-72.

Masilamani, R. 2003. Building a supportive environment for adolescent reproductive health programmes in India: Essential programme components. In S. Bott et al., eds *Towards Adulthood: Exploring the Sexual and Reproductive Health of Adolescents in South Asia:* 156-58. Geneva: World Health Organisation.

Matthews, Z., S. Mahendra, A. Kilaru et al. 2001. Antenatal care, care-seeking and morbidity in rural Karnataka, India: Results of a prospective study. *Asia-Pacific Population Journal*, 16(2): 11-28.

Mavalankar, D.V. 1999a. Human resource management: Issues and challenges. In S. Pachauri, ed., *Implementing a Reproductive Health Agenda in India: The Beginning*. New Delhi: Population Council: 179-200.

Mavalankar, D.V. 1999b. Promoting safe motherhood: Issues and challenges. In S. Pachauri, ed., *Implementing a Reproductive Health Agenda in India: The Beginning*. New Delhi: Population Council: 519-38.

Mavalankar, D. 2002a. Policy and management constraints on access to and use of life-saving emergency obstetric care in India. *Journal of American Medical Women's Association*, 57(3): 165-67.

Mavalankar, D. 2002b. *Report of the Mid-term Review of the Training Component of Reproductive and Child Health Programme of Government of India.* Report submitted to the Training Division, Ministry of Health and Family Welfare, Government of India.

Mavalankar, D. 2003. Maternal health situation in India: Achievements, issues and challenges (unpublished).

Mavalankar, D. and B. Sharma. 1999. The quality of care in sterilization camps: Evidence from Gujarat. In M.A. Koenig and M.E. Khan, eds., *Improving Quality of Care in India's Family Welfare Programme: The Challenge Ahead*: 293-313. New York: Population Council.

Mawar, N., S. Mehendale, S. Thilakavathy et al. 1997. Awareness and knowledge of AIDS and HIV risk among women attending STD clinics in Pune, India. *Indian Journal of Medical Research*, 106: 212-22.

Mayank, S., R. Bahl and N. Bhandari. 2001. Reproductive tract infections in pregnant women in Delhi, India. *International Journal of Gynecology and Obstetrics*, 75: 81-82.

Mayank, S., R. Bahl, A. Rattan et al. 2001. Prevalence and correlates of morbidity in pregnant women in an urban slum of New Delhi. *Asia-Pacific Population Journal*, 16(2): 29-44.

Mehendale, S.M., M.E. Shepherd, A.D. Gangakhedkar et al. 1996. Evidence for high prevalence and rapid transmission of HIV among individuals attending STD clinics in Pune, India. *Indian Journal of Medical Research*, 104:327-35.

Mehra, S., R. Savithri and L. Coutinho. 2002. Sexual behaviour among unmarried adolescents in Delhi, India: Opportunities despite parental controls. Paper presented at the 2002 IUSSP Regional Population Conference, Bangkok, June.

Mehta, R. 2003. Establishing adolescent health services in a general health facility. In S. Bott et al., eds., *Towards Adulthood: Exploring the Sexual and Reproductive Health of Adolescents in South Asia:* 213-18. Geneva: World Health Organisation.

Mehta, A., L. Apers, H. Verstraelen et al. 2001. Trends in caesarean section rates at a maternity hospital in Mumbai, India. *Journal of Health, Population and Nutrition*, 19(4): 306-12.

Mertens, T.E., G.D. Smith, K. Kantharaj et al. 1998. Observations of sexually transmitted disease consultations in India. *Public Health*, 11(2): 123-28.

Ministry of Health and Family Welfare (MOHFW). 1997. *Reproductive and Child Health Programme: Schemes for Implementation*. New Delhi: Government of India.

Ministry of Health and Family Welfare (MOHFW). 1999. *Annual Report, 1998-99*. New Delhi: Government of India.

Ministry of Health and Family Welfare (MOHFW). 2000. *National Population Policy, 2000*. New Delhi: Government of India.

Ministry of Health and Family Welfare (MOHFW). 2002b. *Guidelines for Administration of Emergency Contraceptive Pills by Medical Officers*. New Delhi: MOHFW, Government of India.

Ministry of Health and Family Welfare (MOHFW). 2002b. *India Country Report: Fifth Asian and Pacific Population Conference on "Population and Poverty in Asia and Pacific" Bangkok*. New Delhi, Ministry of Health and Family Welfare, Government of India.

Ministry of Health and Family Welfare (MOHFW). 2003a. *Annual Report, 2002-03*. New Delhi: Government of India.

Ministry of Health and Family Welfare (MOHFW). 2003b. *Family Welfare Programme in India. Year Book 2001*. New Delhi: Department of Family Welfare, MOHFW, Government of India. Available online at: http://health.nic.in.

Ministry of Health and Family Welfare (MOHFW). 2003c. *Family Welfare Programme in India: Introduction*. New Delhi: Department of Family Welfare, Government of India. Available online at: http://health.nic.in.

Ministry of Health and Family Welfare (MOHFW). 2003d. RCH II and Family Planning Programme Implementation Plan (PIP). Draft. Department of Family Welfare, New Delhi: MOHFW, Government of India.

Ministry of Human Resource Development (MHRD). 2001. *National Policy for the Empowerment of Women*. New Delhi: Government of India.

Mishra, U.S. and M. Ramanathan. 2002. Delivery-related complications and determinants of caesarean section rates in India. *Health Policy and Planning*, 17(1): 90-98.

Mishra, D., G. Singh and D. Sharma. 1988. Unsuspected gonococcal infection, candidiasis and trichomoniasis in females. *Indian Journal of Sexually Transmitted Diseases*, 9: 25-28.

Misra, J.S., K. Das and Chandrawati. 2001. Cytological detection of sexually transmitted diseases (STDs) during routine outpatient screening. *Journal of Obstetrics and Gynaecology of India*, 51(4): 133-36.

Misra, J.S., K. Das, P. Tandon et al. 1992. Sexually transmitted pathogens and cervical carcinogenesis. *Journal of Obstetrics and Gynaecology of India*, 42(3): 380-83.

Mondal, A. 1991. Induced abortions in rural society and the need for people's awareness. *Journal of Obstetrics and Gynaecology of India*, 41(4): 450-57.

Mothercare. 1996. Child Survival and Safe Motherhood Programme Review and Assessment: Lessons learned and recommendations: An evaluation report prepared for the Ministry of Health and Family Welfare of India (September-October).

Mukhopadhyay, S. and S. Garimella. 1998. The contours of reproductive choice for poor women: Findings from a micro survey In S. Mukhopadhyay, ed., *Women's Health, Public Policy and Community Action*: 98-121. New Delhi: Manohar.

Mukhopadhyay, C., G. Nath, A.K. Gulati et al. 2001. Prevalence of HIV among low and high risk population of eastern part of northern India. *Journal of Communicable Diseases*, 33(2): 136-42.

Mulgaonkar, V.B. 2001. Childless couples in the slums of Mumbai: An interdisciplinary study. *Asia-Pacific Population Journal*, 16(2): 141-60.

Murthy, N. 1999. The quality of family welfare services in rural Maharashtra: Insights from a client survey. In M.A. Koenig and M.E. Khan, eds., *Improving Quality of Care in India's Family Welfare Programme: The Challenge Ahead*: 33-48. New York: Population Council.

Murthy, N. and A. Barua. 2001. Causes of maternal death in India: A study of contributing factors. Foundation for Research in Health Systems, unpublished report.

Murthy, N., L. Ramachandar, P. Pelto et al. 2002. Dismantling India's contraceptive target system: An overview and three case studies. In N. Haberland and D. Measham, eds., *Responding to Cairo: Case Studies of Changing Practice in Reproductive Health and Family Planning*: 25-57. New York: Population Council.

Muthal-Rathore, A., R. Tripathi and R. Arora. 2002. Domestic violence against pregnant women interviewed at a hospital in New Delhi. *International Journal of Gynaecology and Obstetrics*, 76: 83-85.

Nag, M. 1994. Beliefs and practices about food during pregnancy: Implications for maternal nutrition. *Economic and Political Weekly*, 24(37) (10 September).

Nanda, P. 2002. Gender dimensions of user fees: Implications for women's utilization of health care. *Reproductive Health Matters*, 10(20): 127-34.

Nandan, D., Y.P. Gupta, V. Krishnan et al. 2001. Reproductive tract infection in women of reproductive age group in Sitapur/ Shahjahanpur district of Uttar Pradesh. *Indian Journal of Public Health*, 45(1): 8-13.

Narayana, G. and N. Sangwan. 2001. Implementation of the community needs assessment approach in India. In *Review of Implementation of Community Needs Assessment Approach for Family Welfare in India*. New Delhi: Futures Group International.

Nataraj, S. 1994. Waiting for a connection. *Populi*, 21(10): 6-11.

National AIDS Control Organisation (NACO). 1998. *Country Scenario 1997-98, Government of India.* New Delhi: NACO.

National AIDS Control Organisation (NACO). 2001a. *National Baseline General Population Behavioural Surveillance Survey 2001.* New Delhi: NACO.

National AIDS Control Organisation (NACO). 2001b. *National Baseline High Risk and Bridge Population Behavioural Surveillance Survey 2001: Part 1 Female Sex Workers and their Clients.* New Delhi: NACO.

National AIDS Control Organisation (NACO). 2002a. *National Baseline High Risk and Bridge Population Behavioural Surveillance Survey 2002: Part 2 Men who have Sex with Men and Injecting Drug Users.* New Delhi: NACO.

National AIDS Control Organisation (NACO). 2002b. *National AIDS Prevention and Control Policy.* New Delhi: NACO.

National AIDS Control Organisation (NACO). 2003a. http://www.naco.nic.in

National AIDS Control Organisation (NACO). 2003b. *Flow charts for the Syndromic Management of RTI/STD.* New Delhi: NACO.

National AIDS Control Organisation (NACO) and UNICEF. 2002. Knowledge, attitudes and practices of young adults (15-24 years). New Delhi: NACO and UNICEF.

National Commission on Population. 2002. *Report of the Working Group on Strategies to Address Unmet Needs.* New Delhi: National Commission on Population.

National Crimes Records Bureau. 1995-1999. *Crime in India.* New Delhi: Ministry of Home Affairs.

Neff, D.L. 1994. The social construction of infertility: The case of the Matrilineal Nayars in South India. *Social Science and Medicine*, 39: 475-85.

Nielsen, B.B., J. Liljestrand, M. Hedegaard et al. 1997. Reproductive pattern, perinatal mortality, and sex preference in rural Tamil Nadu, south India: Community-based cross sectional study. *British Journal of Medicine (Clinical Research Ed)*, 314(7093): 1521-24.

Nielsen, B.B., M. Hedgaard, S.H. Thilsted et al. 1998. Does antenatal care influence postpartum health behaviour? Evidence from a community-based cross-sectional study in rural Tamil Nadu, South India. *British Journal of Obstetrics and Gynaecology*, 105(7): 697-703.

Oomman, N. 1996. Poverty and pathology: Comparing rural Rajasthani women's ethnomedical models with biomedical models of reproductive morbidity: Implications for women's health in India. Ph.D Thesis submitted to John Hopkins University, Baltimore.

Oomman, N. 2000. A decade of research on reproductive tract infections and other gynaecological morbidity in India: What we know and what we don't know. In R. Ramasubban and S.J. Jejeebhoy, eds., *Women's Reproductive Health in India*: 236-79. Jaipur: Rawat Publications.

Oomman, N. and B.R. Ganatra. 2002. Sex selection: The systematic elimination of girls. *Reproductive Health Matters*, 10(19): 184-88.

Pachauri, S. 1999. Moving towards reproductive health: Issues and evidence. In S. Pachauri, ed., *Implementing a Reproductive Health Agenda in India: The Beginning*: xiii-xlvii. New Delhi: Population Council.

Pachauri, S. 2000. National Population Policy, 2000: A critique. *Kali's Yug. Women and Law Journal,* March: 19-23.

Pachauri, S. 2001. Implementing population policy: Priorities for Rajasthan. Keynote address at the Conference on 'Issues and Strategies for the Implementation of Population Policy in Rajasthan,' Jaipur, 21-22 December.

Pachauri, S. and A. Jamshedji. 1983. Risks of teenage pregnancy. *Journal of Obstetrics and Gynaecology,* 33(3): 477-82.

Pachauri, S. and K.G. Santhya. 2002a. Reproductive choices for Asian adolescents: A focus on contraceptive behavior. *International Family Planning Perspectives*, 28(4): 186-95.

Pachauri, S. and K.G. Santhya. 2002b. Socio-demographic and reproductive health profile of adolescents in India: A review. *Demography India*, 31(2).

Pachauri, S. and K.G. Santhya. 2003. Contraceptive behaviours among adolescents in Asia: Issues and challenges. In S. Bott et al., eds., *Towards Adulthood: Exploring the Sexual and Reproductive Health of Adolescents in South Asia:* 105-7. Geneva: World Health Organisation.

Pal, A., U.K. Ghosh, G. Ganguli et al. 1993. Socio-demographic profile of sexually transmitted diseases in females. *Journal of Obstetrics and Gynaecology of India*, 43(3): 388-90.

Panda, S., A. Chatterjee, S. Bhattacharjee et al. 1998. HIV, hepatitis B and sexual practices in the street-recruited injecting drug users of Calcutta: Risk perception versus observed risks. *International Journal of STD and AIDS*, 9: 214-18.

Panda, S., U. Saha, S. Pahari et al. 2002. Drug use among the urban poor in Kolkata: Behaviour and environment correlates of low HIV infection. *National Medical Journal of India*, 15(3): 128-34.

Pandit, D.V., R.R. Bhatt, J.M. Karnad et al. 1993. Microbial screening of females with vaginitis. *Journal of Obstetrics and Gynaecology of India*, 43(2): 244-47.

Parashari, A., V. Singh, P. Sodhani et al. 1994. Clinical and aetiological profile of reproductive tract infections (RTIs) among women attending gynaecology out-patient department of a major city hospital in Delhi. *Journal of Obstetrics and Gynaecology of India*, 44(5): 790-97.

Parikh, I., V. Taskar, N. Dharap et al. n.d. Gynaecological morbidity among women in a Bombay slum, unpublished report.

Parivar Seva Sanstha. 1998. *Abortion Research, Phase II: Final Report*. New Delhi: Parivar Seva Sanstha.

Parveen, S., M.E. Khan, J.W. Townsend et al. 1995. *Lesson Learned from a Community-Based Distribution Programme in Rural Bihar*. New Delhi: Population Council.

Patel, T. 1994. *Fertility Behaviour: Population and Society in a Rajasthan Village*. Delhi: Oxford University Press.

Patel, V. 2002. *Gender and Mental Health Research in Developing Countries*. Global Forum for Health Research, November.

Patel, V. and G. Andrew. 2001. Gender, sexual abuse and risk behaviours in adolescents: A cross-sectional survey in schools in Goa. *National Medical Journal of India,* 14(5): 263-67.

Patel, V., M. Rodrigues and N. DeSouza. 2002. Gender, poverty and postnatal depression: A study of mothers in Goa, India. *American Journal of Psychiatry*, 159(1):43-47.

Pelto, P.J. 2000. Research on sexuality and sexual behaviour in India: The 1990s. In R. Ramasubban and S.J. Jejeebhoy, eds., *Women's Reproductive Health in India*: 102-33. Jaipur: Rawat Publications.

Pelto, P.J., A. Joshi and R. Verma. 2000. *Development of Sexuality and Sexual Behaviour among Indian Males: Implications for Reproductive Health Programmes*. New Delhi: Population Council.

Planning Commission. 2001. *Report of the Working Group on Adolescents for the Tenth Five Year Plan (2002-2007)*. New Delhi: Government of India.

Planning Commission. 2002a. *Report of the Steering Committee of Family Welfare*. http://planningcommission.nic.in/aboutus/committee/strgrp/stgp_fmlywel/

Planning Commission. 2002b. *Tenth Five-year Plan, 2002-07*. New Delhi: Government of India.

Poonkhum, Y. 2003. Providing adolescent-friendly reproductive health services: The Thai experience. In S. Bott et al., eds., *Towards Adulthood: Exploring the Sexual and Reproductive Health of Adolescents in South Asia*: 210-12.Geneva: World Health Organisation.

Population Council. 2002. *Cost of Care and Support Services for PLHA: Implications for the Financial Sustainability of Nongovernmental Organizations, Research Summary*. New Delhi: Population Council.

Population Foundation of India and Population Reference Bureau (PFI and PRB). 2003. *HIV/AIDS in India*. New Delhi: Population Foundation of India.

Prabhavathi, K. and S. Sheshadri. 1988. Pattern of IUD use: A follow-up of acceptors in Mysore. *Journal of Family Welfare*, 35(1): 3-16.

Prakasamma, M. 1999a. Andhra Pradesh. In *The Community Need-based Reproductive and Child Health in India: Progress and Constraints*: 18-31. Jaipur: Health Watch Trust.

Prakasamma, M. 1999b. Infertility: A social and gender perspective. Paper presented at the UNFPA Consultation on 'Infertility Prevention and Management,' New Delhi.

Prakasamma, M. 2002. Post-abortion care through the public health system. Paper presented at the Population Council Workshop on 'Abortion in India: How Can Research Help Us Move Forward?' Goa.Prasad, J.H., V. George, M.K. Lalitha et al. 2000. Prevalence of Reproductive Tract Infection among Adolescents in a Rural Community in Tamil Nadu. Paper presented at the workshop on

'Reproductive Health in India: New Evidence and Issues,' Pune, 28 February-1 March.

Puri, C.P. 1998. Contraceptive research and development during the fifty years of independence in India: Achievements and desired goal, *ICMR Bulletin*, 28(10): 89-102.

Qadeer, I. 2000. The National Population Policy: Problems and Possibilities. Paper presented at the Colloquium on National Population Policy 2000, Bangalore, 19-20 October.

Rajaram, N. 2000. Young men's perceptions of their own reproductive health in a slum of Vadodara, unpublished.

Rajaretnam, T. and R.V. Deshpande. 1994. Factors inhibiting the use of reversible contraceptive methods in rural South India. *Studies in Family Planning*, 25(2): 111-21.

Rajgopal, S., A.A. Nagarkar, N.V. Kokate et al. 1989. Foam tablets: An acceptable non-terminal method: Evidence from rural Madhya Pradesh and Tamil Nadu. *Journal of Family Welfare*, 35(4): 3-12.

Ram, K. 1994. Medical management and giving birth: Responses of coastal women in Tamil Nadu. *Reproductive Health Matters*, 4: 20-26.

Rama Rao, S., L. Caleb, M.E Khan et al. 2001. Safer maternal health in rural Uttar Pradesh: Do primary health services contribute? *Health Policy and Planning*, 16(3): 256-63.

Ramachandar, L. 2002. Linking the community and the provider: Village health nurses in Tamil Nadu. Paper presented at the Population Council Workshop on 'Abortion in India: How Can Research Help Us Move Forward?' Goa.

Ramachandar, L. and S. Barge. 1999. The quality of services at laparoscopic sterilization camps in Madhya Pradesh. In M.A. Koenig and M.E. Khan, eds., *Improving Quality of Care in India's Family Welfare Programme: The Challenge Ahead*: 273-92. New York: Population Council.

Ramachandran, P. 1989. Nutrition in pregnancy. In C. Gopalan and S. Kaur, eds., *Women and Nutrition in India*. New Delhi: Nutrition Foundation of India.

Ramakrishna, J., M. Karott and R.S. Murthy. 2003. Experiences of sexual coorcion among street boys in Bangalore, India. In S. Bott et al., eds., *Towards Adulthood: Exploring the Sexual and Reproductive Health of Adolescents in South Asia*: 95-98.Geneva: World Health Organisation.

Ramanathan, M., T.R. Dilip and S.S. Padmadas. 1995. Quality of care in laparoscopic sterilization camps: Observations from Kerala, India, *Reproductive Health Matters*, 6: 84-93.

Ramanathan, M., A. Vijayan, D. Varathrajan et al. 2003. Political decentralization and the primary health care system: Examining the potential for improving women's reproductive health care in Kerala. Paper presented in the National Seminar on 'Global Agendas, Local Realities: Implications of Health Sector Reforms on Woman's Access to Reproductive Health Services in India,' New Delhi, 7 March.

Ramasubban, R. 2000. Women's vulnerability: Recent evidence on sexually transmitted infections. In R. Ramasubban and S.J. Jejeebhoy, eds., *Women's Reproductive Health in India*: 280-330. Jaipur: Rawat Publications.

Ramasubban, R. and B. Rishyasringa. 1998. 'Ashaktapana' (weakness) and reproductive health in a slum population in Mumbai, India. In C.M. Obermeyer, ed., *Cultural Perspectives in Reproductive Health.* Oxford: Oxford University Press.

Ramasubban, R. and B. Rishyasringa. 2000. Treatment seeking by women in Mumbai slums. Paper presented at the workshop on 'Reproductive Health in India: New Evidence and Issues,' Pune, 28 February-1 March.

Rao, A., M. Nag, K. Mishra et al. 1994. Sexual behaviour patterns of truck drivers and their helpers in relation to female sex workers. *Indian Journal of Social Work*, 55(4): 603-15.

Rao, K.S., R.D. Pilli, A.S. Rao et al. 1999. Sexual lifestyle of long distance lorry drivers in India: Questionnaire survey. *British Medical Journal*, 318: 162-63.

Ravindran, T.K.S. 1993. Users' perspective on fertility regulation methods. *Economic and Political Weekly*, 13-20 November:2508-12.

Ravindran, T.K.S. 1995a. *A Study of User Perspectives on the Diaphragm in an Urban Indian Setting.* New Delhi: Rural Women's Social Education Centre and the Population Council.

Ravindran, T.K.S. 1995b. Women's health situation in a rural poor population in Chengalpattu, Tamil Nadu. In M. Das Gupta, L.C. Chen and T.N. Krishnan, eds., *Women's Health in India: Risk and Vulnerabilities*: 175-211. Mumbai: Oxford University Press.

Ravindran, T.K.S. 1999. Rural women's experiences with family welfare services in Tamil Nadu. In M.A. Koenig and M.E. Khan, eds., *Improving Quality of Care in India's Family Welfare Programme: The Challenge Ahead*: 70-91. New York: Population Council.

Registrar General, India (RGI). 1998. *Survey of Causes of Death (Rural): Annual Report 1998.* Series 3, No. 31. New Delhi: Office of the Registrar General.

Registrar General, India (RGI). 1999-2000. *Sample Registration System Estimates*. Office of the Registrar General and Census Commissioner, New Delhi: Planning Commission and Economic Survey.

Registrar General, India (RGI). 2000. *Sample Registration System Bulletin*, April.

Registrar General, India (RGI). 2001. *Census of India, Provisional Population Totals, Series I, Paper I. 2001*. New Delhi: Office of Registrar General.

Retherford, R.D. and T.K. Roy. 2003. Factors affecting sex-selective abortions in India and 17 major states. *National Family Planning Survey Subject Reports, No. 21*. Mumbai: IIPS; Honolulu: East-West Centre.

Risbud, A., K. Chan-Tack, D. Gadkari et al. 1999. The etiology of genital ulcer disease by multiplex polymerase chain reaction and relationship to HIV infection among patients attending sexually transmitted disease clinics in Pune, India. *Sexually Transmitted Diseases*, 26(1): 55-62.

Risbud, A., S. Mehendale, S. Basu et al. 2002. Prevalence and incidence of hepatitis B virus infection in STD clinic attendees in Pune, India. *Sexually Transmitted Infections*, 78(3): 169-73.

Roth, J., S.P. Krishnan and E. Bunch. 2001. Barriers to condom use: Results from a study in Mumbai (Bombay), India. *AIDS Education and Prevention*, 13(1): 65-77.

Row Kavi, A. 1991. Male sex workers: Reaching out. *AIDS Action*, 15:4.

Rowley, J. and S. Berkley. 1998. Sexually transmitted diseases. In C.J.L. Murray and A.D. Lopez, eds., *Health Dimensions of Sex and Reproduction: The Global Burden of Sexually Transmitted Diseases, HIV, Maternal Conditions, Perinatal Disorders, and Congenital Anomalies*: 19-110. Harvard School of Public Health: Harvard University Press.

Roy, T.K and R.K. Verma. 1999. Women's perceptions of the quality of family welfare services in four Indian states. In M.A. Koenig and M.E. Khan, eds., *Improving Quality of Care in India's Family Welfare Programme: The Challenge Ahead*: 19-32. New York: Population Council.

Roy, T.K., D.R. Devi, R.K. Verma et al. 1991. *Health Services and Family Planning in Rural Maharashtra: A Report of the Baseline Survey in Bhandara, Chandrapur, Dhule and Nagpur Districts*, Mumbai: IIPS.

Roy, V., P. Bhargava, J.S. Bapna et al. 1998. Treatment seeking behaviour in sexually transmitted diseases. *Indian Journal of Public Health*, 42(4): 133-35.

Sadhu, S., B.N. Bhattacharya, P.K. Majumdar et al. 2001. Reproductive morbidity among women in weaker sections in Calcutta metropolitan area. *Demography India*, 30(2): 167-91.

Sahasrabuddhe, V.V., T.A. Gholap, Y.S. Jethava et al. 2002. Patient-led partner referral in a district hospital based STD clinic. *Journal of Postgraduate Medicine*, 48(2): 105-8.

Sahi, K. and A. Sarin. 1996. Son factor in family planning acceptance. *Journal of Obstetrics, Gynecology and Family Welfare*, 2(7): 9-13.

Santhya, K.G. 1999. Factors Affecting Reproductive Tract Infections in Southern India. Ph.D. Thesis submitted at Flinders University, South Australia.

Santhya, K.G. 2003. Changing family planning scenario in India: An overview of recent evidence. *Population Council South and East Asia Regional Working Paper No. 17, New Delhi.*

Santhya, K.G. and G.L. Dasvarma. 2002. Spousal communication on reproductive illness among rural women in southern India. *Culture, Health and Sexuality*, 4(2): 223-26.

Santhya, K.G. and S.J. Jejeebhoy. 2003. Sexual and reproductive health needs of married adolescent girls. *Economic and Political Weekly,* 38(41): 4370-77.

Santhya, K.G., E. McGrory and N. Haberland. 2001. First time parents project, Supplemental diagnostic report, Kolkata, unpublished.

Santhya, K.G. N. Haberland, E. McGrory et al. 2003. Supporting married adolescent girls: Encouraging positive partner involvement. Paper presented at the Global Conference on Reaching Men to Improve Reproductive Health for All (September).

Sarkar, S., P. Mookerjee, A. Roy et al. 1991. Descriptive epidemiology of intravenous heroin users: A new risk group for transformation of HIV in India. *Journal of Infection*, 23: 201-7.

Sathyanarayana, K.M. and R. Kar. 2001. Community needs assessment approach for family welfare in Orissa. In *Review of Implementation of Community Needs Assessment Approach for Family Welfare in India.* New Delhi: Futures Group International.

Savara, M. and C.R. Sridhar. 1993. Sexual behaviour patterns amongst men and women in Maharashtra: Results of a survey. Paper presented at the Workshop on 'Sexual Aspects of AIDS/STD Prevention in India,' Mumbai, 23-27 November.

Savara, M. and C.R. Sridhar. 1994. *Report on a Survey of Sexual Behaviour Patterns and Attitudes amongst Men and Women in Maharashtra.* Mumbai: Shakti.

Sebastian, M., D. Huntington, W. Clark et al. 2002a. Project Update 2: Baseline survey results: Integrating adolescent livelihood activities within a reproductive health program for urban slum dwellers in India. New Delhi: Population Council.

Sebastian, M., D. Huntington, B. Mensch et al. 2002b. Project Update 3: Midline survey results: Integrating adolescent livelihood activities within a reproductive health program for urban slum dwellers in India. New Delhi: Population Council.

Sebastian, M.P., D. Huntington, B. Mensch et al. 2003. FRONTIERS final report: Integerating adolescent livelihood activities within a reproductive health program for urban slum dwellers in India, unpublished.

Selvan, M.S., M.W. Ross, A.S. Kapadia et al. 2001. Study of perceived norms, beliefs and intended sexual behaviour among higher secondary school students in India. *AIDS Care*, 13(6): 779-88.

Sen, G., A. Gurumurthy and H. Sudarshan. 1999. Karnataka. In *The Community Need-based Reproductive and Child Health in India: Progress and Constraints*: 75-100. Jaipur: Health Watch Trust.

Senderowitz, J. 1999. Making reproductive health services youth friendly. Washington, D.C.: Pathfinder International, FOCUS on Young Adults.

Sharma, A. and V. Sharma. 1996. Sexual knowledge and practices of college girls in rural Gujarat, India. *Journal of Family Welfare*, 42(3): 19-26.

Sharma, A.K., O.P. Aggarwal and K.K. Dubey. 2002. Sexual behaviour of drug-users: Is it different? *Preventive Medicine*, 34: 512-15.

Sharma, M., N. Nayak, S. Malhotra et al. 1989. Chlamydiazyme test for rapid detection of *Chlamydia trachomatis. Indian Journal of Medical Research,* 89: 4-11.

Sharma, V., S. Dave, A. Sharma et al. 1997. Condoms: Mis-use = non-use: The condom equation in Gujarat, India. *AIDS Care*, 9(6): 707-13.

Sheriar, N.K. 2001. Navigating the MTP Act in clinical practice. *Journal of Obstetrics and Gynaecology of India*, 51: 25-29.

Shrikhande, S.N., S.P. Zodpey and H.R. Kulkarni. 1998. Risk factors and protective factors of pelvic inflammatory disease: A case-control study. *Indian Journal of Public Health*, 42(2): 42-47.

Shrikhande, S.N., S.G. Joshi, S.P. Zodpey et al. 1995. *Chlamydia trachomatis* in pelvic inflammatory disease. *Indian Journal of Pathological Microbiology*, 38(2): 181-84.

Shrivastava, S.P., A. Kumar and A.K. Ojha. 2001. Verbal autopsy determined causes of neonatal deaths. *Indian Paediatrics*, 38:1022-25.

Siddappa, K., V.J. Kumar and K. Ravindra. 1990. Pattern of STDs at Davangere. *Indian Journal of Sexually Transmitted Diseases*, 11: 39-42.

Singh, S. 1998. Adolescent childbearing in developing countries: A global review. *Studies in Family Planning,* 29(2): 117-63.

Singh, A.J. and L.K. Dhaliwal. 1993. Identification of infertile couples in a rural area of northern India. *Indian Journal of Medical Research,* 98: 206-8.

Singh, Y.N. and A.N. Malaviya. 1994. Long distance truck drivers in India: HIV infection and their possible role in disseminating HIV into rural areas. *International Journal of STD and AIDS*, 5: 137-38.

Singh, M. and V.K. Paul. 1997. Maternal and child health services in India with special focus on perinatal services. *Journal of Perinatology,* 17(1): 65-69.

Singh, K.K., S.S. Bloom and A.O. Tsui. 1998. Husband's reproductive health knowledge, attitudes and behaviour in Uttar Pradesh, India. *Studies in Family Planning*, 29(4): 388-99.

Singh, M.M., R. Devi and S.S. Gupta. 1999. Awareness and health seeking behaviour of rural adolescent school girls on menstrual and reproductive health problems. *Indian Journal of Medical Sciences*, 53(9): 439-43.

Singh, A., L.K. Dhaliwal and A. Kaur. 1996. Infertility in A primary health centre of northern India: A follow up study. *Journal of Family Welfare,* 42: 51-56.

Singh, K.G., M.K. Joshi and A.K. Bajaj. 1990. Pattern of sexually transmitted diseases in Allahabad. *Indian Journal of Sexually Transmitted Diseases,* 11: 6-8.

Singh, N.G.B., Y.L. Devi, H.L. Singh et al. 1992. Incidence of HIV (Human immunodeficiency virus) infection and VDRL reactivity among pregnant women. *Journal of Obstetrics and Gynaecology of India*, 42(5): 576-80.

Singh, Y.N., K. Singh, R. Joshi et al. 1993. HIV infection among long distance truck drivers in Delhi, India. *Journal of Acquired Immune Deficiency Syndrome*, 6: 323.

Singh, M.M., R. Devi, S. Garg et al. 2001. Effectiveness of syndromic approach in management of reproductive tract infections in women. *Indian Journal of Medical Sciences,* 55(4): 209-14.

Sinha, G. 1994. The prevalence of wart virus infection and its association with pre-malignant lesions of the cervix. *Journal of Obstetrics and Gynaecology of India*, 44(6): 931-35.

Sinha, R., M.E. Khan, B.C. Patel et al. 1998. Decision-making in acceptance and seeking abortion of unwanted pregnancies. Paper presented at the International Workshop on 'Abortion Facilities and Post-Abortion Care in the Context of the RCH Programme,' New Delhi.

Sodhi, G. and M. Verma. 2003. Sexual coercion amongst unmarried adolescents of an urban slum in India. In S. Bott et al., eds., *Towards Adulthood: Exploring the Sexual and Reproductive Health of Adolescents in South Asia:* 91-94.Geneva: World Health Organisation.

Sodhi, G. and M. Verma. forthcoming. Seeking gratification: A study of sexual behaviour patterns of adolescents in an urban slum. In M. Koenig et al., eds., *Reproductive Health in India: New Evidence.*

Solapurkar, M. and R. Sangam. 1985. Has the MTP Act in India proved beneficial? *Journal of Family Welfare*, 31(3): 46-52.

Solomon, S., N. Kumarasamy, A.K. Ganesh et al. 1998. Prevalence and risk factors of HIV-1 and HIV-2 infection in urban and rural areas in Tamil Nadu, India. *International Journal of STD and AIDS*, 9: 98-193.

Sood, M., Y. Juneja and U. Goyal, 1995. Maternal mortality and morbidity associated with clandestine abortions. *Journal of the Indian Medical Association*, 93(2): 77-79.

Sreevidya, S. and B.W.C. Sathiyasekaran. 2003. High caesarean rates in Madras (India): A population-based cross-sectional study. *British Journal of Obstetrics and Gynaecology*, 110:106-10.

Srikanth, P., T.J. John, H. Jeyakumari et al. 1997. Epidemiological features of acquired immunodeficiency syndrome in southern India. *Indian Journal of Medical Research*, 105:191-97.

Srikantia, S.G. 1989. Pattern of growth and development of Indian girls and body size of adult Indian women. In C. Gopalan and S. Kaur, eds. *Women and Nutrition in India.* New Delhi: Nutrition Foundation of India.

Srinivasa, D.K., K.A. Narayan, A. Oumachigui et al. 1997. *Prevalence of Maternal Morbidity in a South Indian Community*. Pondicherry: Department of Community Medicine, Jawaharlal Institute of Postgraduate Medical Education and Research.

Subba Rao. 2003. School AIDS Education Programme. AP Education Department (presentation).

Sugathan, K.S., V. Mishra and R.D. Retherford. 2001. Promoting institutional deliveries in rural India: The role of antenatal care services. *National Family Health Survey Subject Reports*, No. 20. Mumbai: IIPS.

Thaddeus, S. and D. Maine. 1994. Too far to walk: Maternal mortality in context. *Social Science in Medicine*, 38(8): 1091-1110.

Thomas, K., S.P. Thyagarajan, L. Jeyaseelan et al. 2002. Community prevalence of sexually transmitted diseases and human immunodeficiency virus infection in Tamil Nadu, India: A probability proportional to size cluster survey. *National Medical Journal of India*, 15(3): 135-40.

Times of India. 2002. Abortion-made-easy pill causes alarm in the state, Manjari Mishra, 5 August.

Tuladhar, J.M., J.W. Townsend, N. Haider et al. 1997. Iron supplementation: Knowledge, perceptions and usage among pregnant women in rural India. *Technical Paper* 9, Population Council.

UNESCO. 2000. Cultural settings affect adolescent needs. *Adolescent Education Newsletter*, 3(2): 6.

UNICEF, UNAIDS and WHO. 2002. *Young People and HIV/AIDS: Opportunity in Crisis*. Geneva: United Nations Children's Fund. Joint United Nations Programme on HIV/AIDS, World Health Organisation.

Unisa, S. 1999. Childlessness in Andhra Pradesh, India: Treatment seeking and consequences. *Reproductive Health Matters*, 7: 54-64.

United Nations. 1994. Programme of Action. International Conference on Population and Development.

United Nations. 2001. *World Population Prospects: The 2000 Revision. Volume II: The Sex And Age Distribution of the World Population*. New York: United Nations.

Urmil, A.C., P.K. Dutta, K. Basappa et al. 1989. A study of morbidity patterns among prostitutes attending a municipal clinic in Pune. *Journal of Indian Medical Association*, 87(2): 29-31.

Vajpayee, M., P. Seth and N. Malhotra. 2001. HIV and syphilis in pregnant women at a tertiary hospital. *Tropical Doctor*, 31: 56.

Vajpayee, M., N. Malhotra, P. Seth et al. 2000. HIV seropositivity in women with syphilis in Delhi, India. *Sexually Transmitted Infections*, 76: 59-60.

Varkey, L.C., D. Huntington, A. Das et al. 2001. Involving men in their wives' antenatal and postpartum care in India. Research Update, March New Delhi: Population Council/FRONTIERS.

Venkataramana, C.B.S. and P.V. Sarada. 2001. Extent and speed of spread o HIV infection in India through the commercial sex networks: A perspective. *Tropical Medicine and International Health*, 6(12): 1040-61.

Verma, R.K. and M. Collumbien. 2003. Wife beating and the link with poor sexual health and risk behaviour among men in urban slums in India. *Journal of Comparative Family Studies*, 34(1): 61-74.

Verma, V. and K.B. Das. 1997. Teenage primigravidae: A comparative study. *Indian Journal of Public Health*, 41(2): 52-55.

Verma, R.K and T.K. Roy. 1999. Assessing the quality of family planning service providers in four Indian states. In M.A. Koenig and M.E. Khan, eds., *Improving Quality of Care in India's Family Welfare Programme: The Challenge Ahead*: 169-82. New York: Population Council.

Verma, S., H. Bracken and B. Elul. 2003. Sex-selective abortions in Rajasthan, India, unpublished.

Verma, R.K., G. Rangaiyan, S. Sharma et al. 2000. A study of sexual health problems and treatment seeking behaviour among men in a slum community. Paper presented at the workshop on 'Reproductive Health in India: New Evidence and Issues,' Pune, 28 February-1 March.

Vermuri, M.D. and D. Manohar. 1986. Childlessness in India. *Biology and Society*, 3(4): 163-66.

Vietnam Educational Scientific Institute (VNESI). 1999. Needs assessment study on adolescent reproductive health and behaviours, Bihar. *Population Education Bulletin*, 8(1): 19.

Visaria, L. 1999a. The quality of reproductive health care in Gujarat: Perspectives of female health workers and their clients. In M.A. Koenig and M.E. Khan, eds., *Improving Quality of Care in India's Family Welfare Programme: The Challenge Ahead*: 143-68. New York: Population Council.

Visaria, L. 1999b. Violence against women in India: Evidence from rural Gujarat. *Domestic Violence in India 1: A Summary Report of Three Studies*. Washington, D.C.: International Centre for Research on Women and Centre for Development and Population Activities.

Visaria, L. 2000. From contraceptive targets to informed choice: The Indian experience. In R. Ramasubban and S.J. Jejeebhoy, eds., *Women's Reproductive Health in India:* 331-82. Jaipur: Rawat Publications.

Visaria, L., S.J. Jejeebhoy and T. Merrick. 1999. From family planning to reproductive health: Challenges facing India. *International Family Planning Perspectives,* 25: S44-49.

Visaria, P. and V. Chari. 1998. India's population policy and family planning programme: Yesterday, today and tomorrow. In A. Jain, ed., *Do Population Policies Matter? Fertility and Politics in Egypt, India, Kenya and Mexico*: 53-112. New York: Population Council.

Vishawanath, S., V. Talwar, R. Prasad et al. 2000. Syndromic management of vaginal discharge among women in a reproductive health clinic in India. *Sexually Transmitted Infections,* 76: 303-6.

Viswanathan, H., S. Godfrey and N. Yinger. 1998. *Reaching Women: A Study of Unmet Need in Uttar Pradesh, India*. Washington, D.C.: International Centre for Research on Women.

Watsa, M.C. 1993. Premarital sexual behaviour of urban educated youth in India. Paper presented at the Workshop on Sexual Aspects of AIDS/STD Prevention in India, Mumbai, 23-27 November.

Widge, A. 2001. Beyond natural conception: A sociological investigation of assisted reproduction with special reference to India, Thesis. New Delhi, Jawaharlal Nehru University.

Winikoff, B., I. Sivin, K.J. Coyaji et al. 1997. The acceptability of medical abortion in China, Cuba and India. *International Family Planning Perspectives*, 23: 73-78, 89.

World Bank. 1997. *Project Appraisal Document: India Reproductive and Child Health Project*. World Bank Population and Human Resources Division, South Asia Country Department II, Report # 16393-IN. Washington, D.C.: World Bank.

World Bank. 2000. Reproductive and Child Health Project (RCH) (Cr. N-018)—Mid Term Review Mission, 29 October-17 November. Aide Memoire (unpublished).

World Bank. 2002. *Better Health System for India's Poor: Findings, Analysis, and Options*. Human Development Network; Health, Nutrition and Population Series. Washington, D.C.: World Bank.

World Health Organisation. 1991. Programme on Maternal and Child Health and Family Planning, Division of Family Health, *Infertility: A Tabulation of Available Data on Prevalence of Primary and Secondary Infertility*, WHO/MCH/91.9. Geneva: World Health Organisation.

Zhang, F., A.O. Tsui and C.M. Suchindran. 1999. *The Determinants of Contraceptive Discontinuation in Northern India: A Multilevel Analysis of Calendar Data*. MEASURE Evaluation Project Working Paper. Chapel Hill: Carolina Population Centre, University of North Carolina.

Contributors

Deepika Ganju is a Consulting Editor, and has been associated with social science publications, including books, journals and newsletters as an editor and writer. Her present interests include development-related issues concerning gender, youth, reproductive and sexual health, and water and sanitation. Recently, she has worked closely with the Population Council on a number of projects.

Shireen J. Jejeebhoy, Senior Programme Associate, Population Council, New Delhi, is a demographer involved in social science research on various aspects of sexual and reproductive health. Her particular areas of focus have been gender issues and adolescent sexual and reproductive health and development. Her previous works include *Towards Adulthood: Exploring the Sexual and Reproductive Health of Adolescents in South Asia* (co-edited with Sarah Bott, Iqbal Shah and Chander Puri), *Research Approaches to the Study of Reproductive Tract Infections and Other Gynaecological Morbidities* (co-edited with Michael Koenig and Christopher Elias), *Women's Reproductive Health in India* (co-edited with Radhika Ramasubban) and *Women's Education, Autonomy, and Reproductive Behaviour: Experiences from Developing Countries*.

Vaishali Sharma Mahendra is Senior Programme Officer, Population Council, India. Her work has focused on contextual factors related to HIV/AIDS prevention and care efforts and on issues ranging from stigma and discrimination, sex work, human trafficking and involvement of people living with HIV/AIDS. Her research interests include social and gender equity issues as they relate to preventing and mitigating the impact of the epidemic on women and children and protecting and promoting rights of those infected and affected.

Vijaya Nidadavolu is Communications Specialist in the South and East Asia regional office of the Population Council. Her interests include translating research results into innovative media products and working on strategic communications. She has focused on issues such as domestic violence and more recently on abortion and sex selective abortion.

K.G. Santhya is Senior Programme Officer at the Population Council, New Delhi. Her recent work has focused on designing and testing interventions for married adolescents. She has also worked in other areas including women's reproductive health and ageing. She has published on a variety of topics including STIs/HIV, family planning, adolescent reproductive health, and couple communication.

Mary Sebastian is Programme Officer at the Population Council, New Delhi and is engaged in the Council's programme on adolescents. Her areas of expertise include planning interventions and research for adolescents and women. Prior to joining the Council, she worked with NGOs in implementing intervention programmes and studied the organizational effectiveness of NGOs.

Leila Caleb Varkey is Senior Programme Officer at the Population Council, New Delhi. Her work focuses on operations research relating to health systems, reproductive health services and quality of care. Recently she has coordinated an operations research study focused on involving men in their wives' antenatal and postpartum care and is currently facilitating its scaling-up. Her areas of interest include gender, maternal and child health, male involvement, mother to child transmission of HIV/AIDS, postpartum contraception and urban health.

Ravi K. Verma is Programme Associate, Population Council, New Delhi. His areas of interest include sexuality, sexual behaviour and male sexual health issues from the viewpoint of HIV/AIDS prevention and care; youth, reproductive health and capacity building. He was on the faculty of the International Institute for Population Sciences (IIPS), Mumbai for over two decades before joining the Population Council. His previous work includes the publication of a co-edited volume entitled *Sexuality in the Times of AIDS: Contemporary Perspectives from Communities in India*.

Shalini Verma is currently a Senior Research Manager at TNS India. Earlier she was a Research Officer at the Population Council, New Delhi where she worked on abortion-related research. Her interests and previous work focus on such reproductive health issues as HIV/AIDS, sex selective abortion and abortion.

Anjali Widge is currently a Research Fellow at the Centre for Population Studies, London School of Hygiene and Tropical Medicine, University of London. Earlier, she was a Programme Officer at the Population Council, New Delhi. Her research has focused on the socio-cultural implications of reproductive technologies, specifically assisted reproduction, women's reproductive health, women's work in the informal sector and adolescents' livelihood related issues. Currently she is exploring women's experiences with infertility services in India.

Index